Quality in Audiology: Design and Implementation of the Patient Experience

Editor-in-Chief for Audiology
Brad A. Stach, PhD

Quality in Audiology: Design and Implementation of the Patient Experience

Brian Taylor, AuD

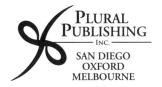

PLURAL
PUBLISHING
INC.
SAN DIEGO
OXFORD
MELBOURNE

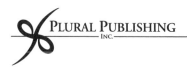

5521 Ruffin Road
San Diego, CA 92123

e-mail: info@pluralpublishing.com
Web site: http://www.pluralpublishing.com

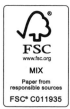

FSC
www.fsc.org
MIX
Paper from
responsible sources
FSC® C011935

Typeset in 11/13 Garamond by Flanagan's Publishing Services, Inc.
Printed in the United States of America by McNaughton & Gunn, Inc.

Library of Congress Cataloging-in-Publication Data

Taylor, Brian, 1966-
  Quality in audiology: design and implementation of the patient
experience / Brian Taylor.
      p. ; cm.
  Includes bibliographical references and index.
  ISBN-13: 978-1-59756-472-4 (alk. paper)
  ISBN-10: 1-59756-472-9 (alk. paper)
  I. Title.
  [DNLM: 1. Audiology. 2. Hearing Aids. 3. Practice Management—
organization & administration. 4. Quality of Health Care. WV 270]
  RF290
  617.8—dc23
                                                    2013006765

CONTENTS

INTRODUCTION

"Ch-ch-ch-ch-changes. Turn and face the strange . . . " That is what David Bowie told us in 1971, and oddly enough, it is an accurate way to summarize what is happening with health care. If you have been paying attention for the past few years, you have noticed many changes in the delivery of health care services. In fits and starts, physicians and other allied health professionals are beginning to be reimbursed for the quality of their results, rather than the sheer number of procedures they order. Hospitals and clinics that demonstrate higher-than-average patient satisfaction scores are enjoying higher rates of reimbursement from federally funded programs. Patients are joining the quality bandwagon as many are demanding greater transparency when shopping for medical services. Consumer-centered health care is gradually supplanting the antiquated, paternalistic model in which the practitioner is never questioned and has near omnipotent authority over the uninformed patient. Out of this paradigm shift comes the quality movement. For audiologists this means the use of report cards, key performance indicators, and other quality strategies and tactics, if they want to stay relevant in a highly competitive marketplace. If you are like the typical practitioner, there is a good chance these concepts related to quality are strange to you now, but they will not be after you read this book.

TOP-DOWN AND BOTTOM-UP QUALITY

There is no shortage of boards, institutions, and organizations that have defined and implemented quality standards. Hearing aid manufacturers are required to follow the certification processes of the International Standardization Organization (ISO) if they expect to stay competitive. Physicians and other medical professionals are credentialed through the National Committee for Quality Assurance (NCQA), which is an independent organization designed to improve the quality of health care through voluntary accreditation and reporting of outcomes. Beginning in October 2013, eligible hospitals will be required to report clinical quality measures for incentive payments. Even audiologists can participate in the quality movement through reporting various clinical procedures completed on patients to the Physician Quality Reporting System (PQRS), which is a program administered through the Centers for Medicare and Medicaid Services (CMS). The American Academy of Audiology (AAA), Academy of Doctors of Audiology (ADA), and American Speech and Hearing Association (ASHA) are quite active in the quality movement. This type of "top-down" push for quality by these organizations is definitely a good thing for everyone, but as this book attempts to demonstrate, the push for better quality starts within the trenches of the audiologist's clinic.

This book is not about how these important agencies and governing bodies hold professionals accountable and protect the well-being of consumers by mandating processes and standards designed to improve quality. That task is left in the capable hands of the quality control leaders of these groups. Of course, all of these initiatives established by these groups are critical to the long-term success of the profession of audiology and the hearing aid industry. As health care becomes more consumer-centric, these standardization agencies will continue to wield more influence over the daily work of the clinician. In an age of transparency this is simply a fact of life. The problem, however, is that the workaday practitioner is easily overwhelmed and unnecessarily burdened with the "bureaucracy of quality." This is unfortunate because the essence of quality resides in the thoughtful actions of the individual clinician who spends hundreds of hours per year face-to-face with patients.

The purpose of this book is to bring practical tools surrounding quality to life for the average clinician who must defend the value of their services to patients. Quality is improved mainly through your grassroots initiatives: procedures, programs, and *behaviors* you implement, measure, and manage in your clinic. This grassroots perspective requires audiologists and other professionals associated with hearing heath care to reexamine the concept of quality. According to ISO, quality is the totality of characteristics, including people, processes, products environments, standards, and learning, of an entity that bear upon its ability to satisfy stated and implied needs. This definition suggests we improve ourselves and our ability to create quality in the world around us through innovation and the judicious use of best practice standards.

From a workaday, clinical standpoint, quality is meeting the requirements and expectations of patients *and* stakeholders in the business. (A stakeholder is defined as anyone who receives payment for their direct work in the business.) In short, quality is probably best defined as the standardization of individual excellence. Rather than rely on academic boards and government agencies, the quest for better quality begins with self-motivated and dedicated audiologists and support staff who can implement many of the concepts and tactics presented in this book.

One of the key points of this book is that the business of audiology is a blend of a medical and a retail model. We are a little of Mayo Clinic and a little of Nordstrom, but not completely similar to either of these very respected enterprise's business models. This unique merger of the medical and commercial sectors has a profound effect on quality.

LESSONS FROM BUSINESS

More than 10 years ago, Jim Collins, a former professor from the Stanford University Graduate School of Business, wrote one of the most widely read business books of all time. *Good to Great: Why Some Companies Make the Leap . . . and Others Don't* describes how average companies are transformed into great companies. "Great" is defined as financial performance several times better than the market average over a sustained period of time, and, as Chapter 5 illustrates, it is one component of quality. Collins' analysis uncovered seven characteristics that differentiate a great company from one that is merely good. These seven characteristics include:

- Level 5 Leadership—humble yet driven leaders who act in the best interest of the company
- First Who, Then What—finding and hiring people who are the right fit for your business
- Confront the Brutal Facts—confronting the cold, hard truth while simultaneously maintaining optimism about the performance of your business
- Hedgehog Concept—identifying something about which you are passionate and which you can make money doing, and then try to be the best in the world at doing it
- Culture of Discipline—executing on the mundane and ordinary details of your business
- Technology Acceleration—using technology to accelerate growth of your company
- The Flywheel—leveraging the additive effect of many small projects and initiatives that are all geared to generate more revenue for your business

In 2001, when the book was published, 11 businesses made the "great list." Today, a couple of these great companies no longer exist, and another eight are actually underperforming compared with the most recent Standards and Poor 500 index. Many books, like *Good to Great*, do an outstanding job of *what* needs to get done. This book, on the other hand, attempts to show you *how* and *why*.

Good to Great and other books like it give mostly a look at past performance. As we all know, the future is impossible to predict; however, the present book will give you the tools to prepare for it. What made your business successful 2 years ago may no longer be effective. Although a book like *Good to Great* may help unravel some knotty management problems, it is probably not going to help redefine certain parameters of your business or clinic as competitive landscapes and technology evolve and quality becomes central to long-term success.

If we cannot rely on best-selling business books to provide us with new ideas, where can we turn? A good start might be the ancient Greeks. Aristotle came up with the idea of practical wisdom (phronesis). The Greeks defined practical wisdom as the ability to consider the mode of action to deliver change, especially to enhance quality of life in the real world. When you look around, there are all kinds of examples of how practical wisdom can be applied to everyday business and clinical situations. The military, science, sports, and the arts provide us with several inspirational examples of practical wisdom. One example can be found in the work of Eric Greitens, a U.S. Navy Seal. His story of humanitarian relief efforts in the war-torn Middle East holds immense lessons for any owner, manager, or clinician concerned about quality and an individual's commitment to excellence. His basic message is that it takes a lot of personal courage (a willingness to stand up and fight for what you believe is right, even in the face of opposing popular opinion) and teamwork to overcome life's obstacles. As you are sure to learn by reading this book, quality is incrementally improved only through the courage to have a sustained personal commitment to excellence.

LESSONS FROM MEDICINE

Another source for practical wisdom and a personal commitment to excellence comes from the work of Dr. Atul Gawande, a Boston-area physician and best-selling author. If you are looking for timeless ways to transform your practice through quality, apply a dose of his practical wisdom. Dr. Gawande's approach to the delivery of medical care represents several "best practices" that audiologists would be wise to replicate in their clinics. These best practices include the following:

- Ask unscripted questions of patients and be an active listener. This is an attempt to make our busy world seem a little more human. You never know when that 95-year-old patient who is struggling with their hearing aids was once a famous classically trained pianist during World War II.
- Do not complain. As a keen observer of world events, you might think there are plenty of things about which to be unhappy, but there is nothing more dispiriting than

being around highly trained professionals who like to carp about things they do not like. The world can be a pretty dreary place when there is too much complaining, so find something positive about which to talk. It could be the last book you read or the TV show you watched last night. Whatever it is, change the subject and do not fall into the trap of being a chronic complainer.

- Measure something. Audiology is a field founded on scientific principles. All of us had to have some background in science in order to get a degree. Take the time to measure something in your practice. It could be number of appointments scheduled, number of hearing aids dispensed per month, or real-world outcomes of your hearing aid fittings. As you will read, by measuring something you begin the process of improving it.

This book places quality in the context of the patient's experience in your clinic. There are six distinct interaction stations that serve as the stage for implementing and improving quality. In practical terms, this engaging patient experience is nothing more than your ability to customize the delivery of products and services for the individual patient around a dominating principle. Quality is that dominating principle. Some of the core components of quality, as you will read, include clarity of purpose, discipline in specific actions, and an ability to emotionally connect with patients and staff.

Kaizen is a Japanese word that means continuous improvement. (The Japanese are responsible for many of the quality concepts discussed here.) *Kaizen*, like quality, is something that everyone can agree is important. The reality is that very few organizations and individuals fully embrace the principles of *kaizen*. Most individuals simply leave it to chance and proclaim that they are improving all the time. They may be attending a course, reading a book, or networking with other professionals. These endeavors may be helpful on the surface, but it is the *way* that organizations and individuals make improvements that really matters.

When *kaizen* and quality are truly embraced, the bulk of improvement is done by people who actually do the work, not the boards or agencies that establish the standards. Using the six patient-experience interactions as the foundation, this book will show you how to become deeply engaged with patients and staff so that quality can be continuously improved. In the end, it is the front office professional and clinician, both of whom connect with patients every day, not the expert, absentee manager, or consultant, who must put quality into action.

Quality is something about which everyone, from the military to musicians, needs to be concerned. To borrow a lyric from the British rock group, The Clash, "Don't you ever stop long enough to start." Professionals dedicated to excellence must never stop thinking about new ways of putting quality into action. Let us hope you embrace the concepts in this book avidly enough to start an ongoing dialogue with your colleagues about quality. It is time to practice audiology differently. You can start by reading this book. The future of your profession depends on it.

1

QUALITY AND THE PATIENT EXPERIENCE

Love, despair, and quality are some of the terms used to describe the human condition. They are experienced by everyone, yet a clear definition of each remains elusive. Most of us innately know what these conditions feel like, but for many of us, these concepts are almost indefinable. There are, of course, examples of quality in both the delivery of health care and the management of a business. This book addresses quality in both of them. To truly understand quality, however, we must think more precisely about its definition. Most of us can describe a restaurant known for the quality of its food and service. We know what to expect from a pair of high-quality shoes. Some of us might even know what it is like to drive a high-quality sports car. Each of us can probably describe the difference between high and low quality for important or meaningful aspects of our lives, but the real challenge is in instilling a desire for quality in our profession and in our business. In a world surrounded by relatively high-quality products, a passion for delivering a high-quality service experience may be the next frontier in health care. Like politics, religion, and sex, quality of care is not a polite topic of conversation among friendly audiologists. It is nearly taboo to

1

discuss the merits of good-quality delivery of services. This book intends to change this.

The primary purpose of this book is to more precisely define quality and bring the concept to life in our practices in the delivery of hearing care to patients. When we take the courageous step of trying to define and measure quality, we not only can better understand it, but can also have the ability to transform our profession and our business. By implementing the concepts and tactics presented in this book, audiologists can successfully differentiate their service offerings to the marketplace of hearing-impaired individuals, while simultaneously raising the overall level of care provided to these patients. As you will learn, delivering a high-quality service experience is just the beginning. Quality is a very broadly defined term that addresses everything from product reliability to marketing campaigns. Everything from the workflow of your office to the final outcome of the hearing aid fitting is part of quality. Quality is the common thread between all the links in your practice from the front office scheduling to the back office accounting. Although this book certainly does not have all the answers in the quest to fully understand all there is to know about quality in an audiology practice, it will get you on the path to defining and improving quality in your practice. Along with providing the reader with a clearer definition of quality, this book will also provide you with some tools to measure and improve several facets of quality.

In order to more fully understand the importance that quality has in the delivery of hearing care, let us place quality in some historical context. Over a relatively short period of time, more than 30 years ago, important contributions to the field were made by pioneers such as Raymond Carhart, Sam Lybarger, Cy Libby, and many others. Due mainly to the work of these pioneers, audiology went from a fledging cottage industry to an independent profession within the course of about two decades. No work better encapsulates this transition from a pre-World War II backwaters subject to a thriving profession than that of James Jerger. In order to better appreciate both the breadth and depth of Jerger's work, the reader is referred to his book, *Clinical Audiology: The Jerger Perspective*, published in 1993. This book is a tribute to Jerger's legacy as a collaborative scientist and influential teacher who spearheaded the creation of a profession. Reading his book 20 years after it was published also sheds light on the new challenges audiologists face in the second decade of the 21st century. Now is the time for a new generation of professionals to breathe life into audiology by raising the bar on how it is systematically practiced. Seizing on quality initiatives is part of this endeavor. As with other health sciences, audiologists have access to an impressive array of modern tests and automated digital algorithms. We have the ability to accurately and quickly assess the entire auditory system for newborns to geriatrics. What seems to be missing is a collective ability to standardize clinical processes in a manner that leads to better patient care, better outcomes, and more profitable business. Historically, standardized clinical processes, evidence-based decision making and best practices have been touted by audiologists in academia and largely ignored by the practitioner. This books attempts to change this dichotomy. By centering clinical processes and business practices around quality, this book attempts to move the work of the audiology pioneers as well as that of the clinicians of today to a new level of patient care that is recognized by the public as comprehensive and exceptional: a level of patient care excellence grounded in quality.

Audiologists live in an interconnected world. Gone are the heady days when a profession could focus exclusively on the science of the auditory system or amplification devices and continue to be a viable profession. In order to have a sustainable business model, audiologists must embrace the science as well as the art of delivering outstanding patient care. In an era of evidence-based medicine in which patients have a choice where they spend their hard-earned dollars, both the science and the art are critically important. Audiologists must appreciate the work of Jerger and others. Their pioneering efforts have made the practice of audiology a worthwhile business opportunity. Audiologists need to build upon the legacy of these pioneers by embracing quality, which, in the broadest sense of the term, is a concept that touches on both the clinical and business side of the equation. As you will learn, quality is an art, but it is mainly a science. The role quality plays in the management of an audiology practice requires us to think differently about how we delivery services to patients. We must first acknowledge that consumers have a choice in how they spend their time and money and patients have a right to experience innovative and comprehensive care. In the digital era, where consumers have access to a wide range of effective technology, the path to success revolves around delivering a memorable patient experience. At the heart of delivering this memorable and remarkable patient experience is the clinician's ability to focus on quality.

In today's era of disruptive innovation and economic uncertainty, there are an abundance of challenges facing many hearing aid dispensing practices. Regardless of your business model, these challenges are likely to include keeping pace with new hearing aid technology, hiring the right staff, and maintaining a profitable business. Among the major obstacles many practices face on a daily basis is the finite number of prospects willing to consider their product and service offerings. This chapter sheds light on the challenge of bringing prospects to your clinic in an era in which traditional marketing mediums are losing their effectiveness and consumers have available to them a vast array of choices.

For various reasons the industry has been plagued with an inability to convert qualified leads into loyal patients. (A lead, sometimes called an opportunity, is defined as a person who has an aidable hearing loss who seeks your services.) First, relative to other medical professions, the market for hearing aid services is relatively small. Consider that approximately 16% of adults in the U.S. suffer from hearing loss (Agrawal, Platz, & Niparko, 2008). Furthermore, of the 26 million Americans who have significant hearing loss, 17.9 million do not want or need amplification. This suggests that the untapped market for hearing aids is about 8 million individuals, suggesting a 51.3% market penetration rate (Amlani & Taylor, 2012). Among the non-owners of amplification some will be in denial for the proverbial 7 to 10 years, whereas others in this group refuse to try hearing aids because of stigma or because they simply cannot afford them. In short, the footprint (defined as the number of prospects within a 20- to 30-min commute to your business) of any given practice often attracts less than 100 motivated hearing-impaired individuals over a 120- to 150-day window of time. Given the abundance of options available to the relatively small number of consumers in need of amplification, and the growing number of options available to purchase amplification devices and related services, such as the

Internet, mail order, and other direct-to-consumer options, hearing care professionals must find more effective ways to differentiate their offerings in an increasingly crowded marketplace.

A second set of challenges facing hearing care professionals of all stripes is related to the use of common business and clinical practices. For example, we know that once a motivated hearing-impaired prospect inquires about products and services many practices are faced with a litany of potential landmines that can diminish the overall productivity of their business, not to mention the final outcome of the fitting. Among these landmines are:

- An inability to schedule appointments for prospects inquiring about services.
- An inability to convert qualified prospects into hearing aid users (Taylor, 2009).
- A combined in-the-drawer, return for credit, and low daily use rate of 30% (Kochkin, 2009).
- Lower than expected benefit from patients who experience a minimalist clinical protocol (Kochkin et al., 2010).

Most of us would agree there are opportunities for improvement. What makes these statistics more perilous, however, is that a couple of different societal trends do not favor the traditional patient–provider service delivery model. Over the past 5 to 10 years two gradual societal transformations, one involving technology and the other relating to consumer behavior, have occurred. These slow-moving societal transformations have occurred largely beyond the purview of the hearing care community.

The first transformation is related to the increasing availability of over-the-counter personal sound amplification products (PSAPs). Due to a loophole in the FDA regulations, PSAPs, which are devices that are designed to "enhance communication" for recreational or workplace activities for persons with normal hearing, are allowed to mingle in the traditional hearing aid market. Although PSAPs and other similar over-the-counter-type devices have been available for quite some time, it is only relatively recently that they have become available through third-party insurance providers and so-called big-box electronic outlets.

THE AGE OF DISRUPTIVE
INNOVATION AND OUTSOURCING

PSAPs as well as other types of direct-to-consumer devices represent a growing trend in disruptive innovation that has challenged virtually every industry at one time or another since the Industrial Revolution. Recently, however, the combination of low-cost electronics combined with the Internet has enabled disruptive innovations to challenge many elective medical procedure markets, including hearing aids.

According to Christensen (2003) there are two types of disruptive innovations. Low-end disruptions target customers who do not need or desire to have the full performance valued by customers already using the product or technology. Low-end disruption commonly overtakes a traditional product or technology when the rate at which the product improves exceeds the rate at which customers can adapt to new performance features. Low-cost cameras and laptop computers with limited features are two prime examples of low-end disruptive technology.

The second type of disruptive innovation is new market disruption. This occurs when the needs of a specific group of customers go underserved for a prolonged period of time; thus, a new and often less expensive technology can capture untapped sectors of the market. The Sony pocket radio, for example, introduced a large group of teenagers who could not afford, or lacked the space for, a tabletop radio to the pleasures rock-and-roll in the late 1950s.

Over-the-counter PSAPs represent both low-end and new market disruptions. Given the relatively low market penetration rates of hearing aid adaptation, 30% "failure rate," and cost barriers associated with hearing aid use for some individuals, audiologists need to understand and potentially find ways to unleash the power of disruptive technology in their practices to grow their business without cannibalizing their existing core patient base.

Disruptive innovations are certainly not confined to products. The outsourcing of medical procedures to developing nations, such as India or China, represents another threat to the future of audiology and hearing aid dispensing as it has been traditionally practiced. Other medical professions, such as radiology, have already felt the impact of medical outsourcing. It is not too difficult to imagine a day when hearing aids are remotely fitted and fine-tuned from an office halfway across the world by audiologists or hearing instrument specialists paid a fraction of the cost of their North American counterparts.

Hearing care professionals can begin the process of embracing disruptive innovations through a better understanding of quality and how to bring various "quality initiatives" to life in their clinics. As you will learn, a critical component to quality is using a data-driven approach to answering questions and solving problems. In the particular example below, audiologists can use data to segment their market.

Traditionally, market segmentation involves compartmentalizing patients based on age, degree of hearing loss, or income. Once segmented along age, hearing loss, or income, audiologists can devise marketing strategies to reach various segments of the market. To leverage the concept of disruptive innovation, however, audiologists must segment their patients in a different way. By asking the question, *What jobs do hearing-impaired patients hire me to do?*, audiologists can begin to better understand the role disruptive innovations might have in their practice. The answer to this important question often leads to one of two possible unexpected answers:

- A no-frills product without service support.
- An experience. Expert advice, outstanding service, and emotional engagement wrapped around a customized electronic medical device.

Both of these unexpected answers may lead audiologists to offer products, services, and experiences to an underserved segment of their market. In the case of a no-frills product, it may lead audiologists to offer an over-the-counter device as a sort of starter hearing aid. In terms of an experience, it may encourage the audiologist to enhance the overall quality of the relationship with patients during their journey through the clinic.

Another phenomenon associated with disruptive innovation is the outsourcing of medical procedures. Due to high-speed Internet connections, Skype, and other types of technology, academically trained professionals can conduct the reading of test results from remote locations; thus, highly trained medical professionals can reside in a location where they are paid the going rate for their services while completing these tasks at a fraction of the cost. In addition to the remote reading of test results, experts tell us that robotic surgery is on the horizon. For the hearing care professional, the emergence of this type of outsourcing may take the form of tele-audiometry in which the work of several clinicians is completed remotely by computer-based audiometers that are overseen by a single audiologist who may reside in a remote location.

@CONNECT

Clayton Christensen

Clayton Christensen is the Kim B. Clark Professor of Business Administration at the Harvard Business School, where he teaches one of the most popular elective classes for second-year students, Building and Sustaining a Successful Enterprise. He is regarded as one of the world's top experts on innovation and growth, and his ideas have been widely used in industries and organizations throughout the world. His first book, *The Innovator's Dilemma*, received the Global Business Book Award as the best business book of 1997. In 2011 *The Economist* named it as one of the six most important books about business ever written.

THE HEALTHY AGING MOVEMENT IN AN ERA OF MINDFUL SPENDING

Over the past decade the American economy has undergone upheaval on a seismic scale, unlike any time since the Great Depression. There is evidence suggesting that the current economic uncertainty is the new normal and that it has begun to systematically change the buying habits and priorities of many consumers (Benett & O'Reilly, 2010). Benett and O'Reilly present evidence, gathered from more than 7,000 consumers, that consumer buying habits are undergoing a shift away from gratuitous consumption to more mindful spending. This paradigm shift in consumer behavior, which certainly could have an effect on how individuals approach the hearing aid market, can be broken down into five distinct ways the "new consumer" is approaching the market:

- Embracing Substance—A growing number of consumers are disenchanted with the buying transaction. They are looking for a reason to connect with a product or service. The "new consumer" is craving real, authentic experiences, and they are willing to hang on to their cash until they feel a sense of engagement with a product, service, or business.
- Rightsizing—Many consumers feel paralyzed with the sheer number of choices for any given product. They are seeking a move toward simplification in which a trusted family member, friend, or other influencer is able to help them make an intelligent decision.
- Growing Up—Nearly everyone has been personally touched by unemployment from the recent economic malaise or family upheaval resulting from a decade of low-intensity war in the Middle East. The result of this is a movement beyond immediate gratification and a trend toward establishing a sense of community with others, including businesses.
- Seeking Pleasure with a Purpose—Impulse shopping is losing its sense of appeal with the "new consumer." People are still willing to spend money, but the trend is toward a more conscientious form of consumption in which shoppers do their homework, and seek to connect and establish a long-term relationship with businesses that have the same values as theirs.
- Living Well, Not Aging Gracefully—It has been said that people born after the year 1945 want to live to be 100

in the body of someone who looks and feels 50. Healthy Agers are often interested in tools (i.e, coaches, medicines, alternative therapies, etc.) that will enable them to look and feel youthful. The role of the Audiologist is to supply this knowledge and information to Healthy Agers as they continue to live well—even into their 90s and beyond.

Data from Benett and O'Reilly (2010) suggest that Healthy Agers are often looking for businesses to replace the personal relationships of family or friends that might be residing in other locations. Additionally, Healthy Agers are choosing to forego retirement, work past the age of 70 years, and even begin a new career. Given the different needs of Healthy Agers coupled with the fact that they represent a significant portion of future business, hearing health professionals must learn as much as possible about what makes this group tick in order to meet their demands for quality.

#DISCOVER

Your first lesson about quality is that it is process oriented. The patient-experience cycle is a process in which quality can be continuously improved through the design, implementation, and measurement at each of the six interaction stations.

THE CHALLENGE OF LIMITED CAPACITY: THE ONE QUESTION YOU MUST ASK YOURSELF

Time is the most precious resource for all of us. With a finite number of working hours in a day, audiologists must prioritize how their time is allotted. Although it would be advantageous to attract all segments of the hearing aid market to your clinic, the reality is that we cannot meet the needs of all segments of the market, especially new markets that disruptive innovations may open.

You can build your business around one segment of the market by asking one simple question, "What do I want to be known for in my marketplace?" The answer to this question will enable you to build a business around one tangible characteristic of a product or service that appeals to consumers. Being known as the leader in one of these segments often gives you the distinct privilege of commanding a higher average selling price or garnering more free word-of-mouth advertising. Here are the four possible answers to this question, which get at the heart of what customers are willing to purchase:

- Price—Like Wal-Mart you are known for charging the lowest prices. The segment of the market looking for no frills and low quality will seek you. Before embracing this model, remember that low prices can be easily matched.
- Convenience—Like McDonald's you are known for easy access and predictability. Like low-price leaders, convenience leaders offer no frills and this can be easily matched by tools such as the Internet.
- Technology—Like Apple you are known for offering innovative and cool gadgets. The downside to adapting this model in the hearing aid business is that everyone is offering essentially the same products. Additionally, consumers expect that technology will continue to evolve and improve.
- The Experience—The "progression of economic value" (Pine & Gilmore, 2011) suggests that when you move beyond price, convenience, and technology to provide a memorable and emotionally engaging experience, you can attract consumers to your practice who are willing to pay a premium for the opportunity to be transformed. From the consumer segmentation point of view, the audiologist's ability to provide this memorable and remarkable experience has tremendous potential to drive the overall productivity of any audiology practice willing to put the business model into place. Next, let us build a case for why practices must embrace the experience-based business model.

@*CONNECT*

Joe Pine

To learn more about the importance of providing a memorable patient experience and the progression of economic value, see the Pine and Gilmore book, *The Experience Economy.* To learn more follow Joe Pine @joepine.

ORCHESTRATING QUALITY THROUGH THE PATIENT JOURNEY

Let us get right into the practical application of quality by examining the patient journey and how it relates to quality. We can do this by examining something that nearly everyone does several times per year: a visit to your favorite restaurant. Even though all of us define a "high-quality" meal differently, there are some commonalities that separate a restaurant known for quality regardless of its location, type of food, and prices. All of us have a certain set of expectations we think about when we patron our favorite restaurant. We expect it to be clean, to have comfortable seating, friendly and prompt service, and great-tasting food, among other attributes. The best restaurants are able to sequence the customer's "journey" through the restaurant, orchestrate staff to play a specific role during each phase of this journey, follow certain standards in order for the entire staff to work together to bring you a consistently good meal, and, finally, an ability to elicit your feedback so that they can improve quality incrementally over time, so that the restaurant continues to meet your ever-changing needs and desires. Delivering quality in a clinical practice functions in essentially the same way. It starts with our ability to sequence or orchestrate a series of events we often call the "patient journey." Let us take a closer look at the sequencing of events within your office and how this contributes to quality.

Many audiologists have been trained such that the patient's "journey" through a clinic can be classified into three appointments: (1) prefitting, (2) fitting, and (3) follow-up. The prefitting appointment is typically a series of audiometric tests, case history, and needs assessment that determines hearing aid candidacy. The fitting appointment is a series of steps, usually involving hearing aid software, in which the professional sets the stage for initial hearing aid use and ensures the fitting is meeting some predefined standard. Finally, there is a series of two to four follow-up appointments in which fine-tuning and additionally counseling are delivered by the clinicians. Although each of these appointments is necessary, viewing the patient–clinician interaction in this manner is a very professional-centric point of view. Since quality is a patient-centric concept, perhaps there is a better way to portray this interaction. Moreover, many audiologists would agree that the way patients interact with your practice has undergone a remarkable transition over the past 3 to 5 years. Patients simply have more choices when it comes to hearing care services. Gone are the days when you could post an occasional promotional offer in your local newspaper and generate immediate sales. The question is, what ought I be doing differently to overcome the effects of these changes to the marketplace? The answer starts with sequencing the patient journey and turning the entire process into a memorable experience for the patient.

Finally, we know that a key to overcoming the uncertainty of disruptive technology and alternative distribution models is through differentiation of your practice. One way to be different is to make the patient's interaction with your practice so memorable and enjoyable that individuals flock to your door seeking a transformative, life-changing event delivered by you. By enhancing the patient's interaction with your practice at these six critical areas of interaction (Figure 1–1), you can begin to unlock the secrets of a truly transformative experience for your patient while commanding a higher average selling price. Later in this chapter we discuss a quality methodology called Six Sigma. An important component of Six Sigma is something called the "value stream" which is more or less a sequence of steps that transform raw materials into a commercial product for which a customer is willing to pay. Although Figure 1–1 does not look like a stream, the process steps shown are designed to transform information, products, and services into a sellable product for which hearing-impaired patients are willing to pay.

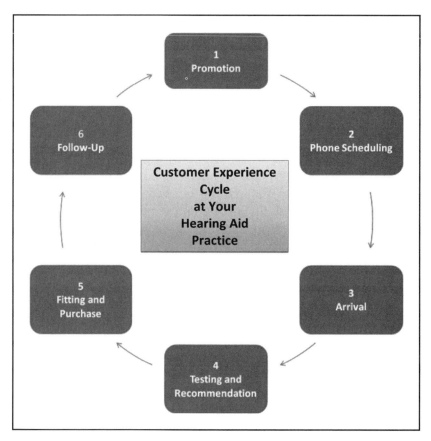

Figure 1–1. The six patient–provider interaction stations or value stream.

Perhaps more importantly, sequencing the patient journey is also a way to begin the process of systematizing the critical points of contact between the audiologist and patient. By demarcating a finite series of specific interaction points, we can orchestrate what needs to occur at each point, develop standards of care for each point, and define a success outcome for each point. Figure 1–1 shows six distinct points of contact with a patient in a hearing aid dispensing practice. For each point of contact very specific processes can be created. Predefined standards, which are often best practice guidelines, can be used to ensure that each sequence leads to a successful outcome. By sequencing the patient journey using best practices, it is more

---

#DISCOVER

Best Practices

Throughout this book you will see the term "best practices." Probably the best way to define the term is to say that best practices are a method or technique that has consistently shown results superior to those achieved with other means. Best practices are used to maintain quality as an alternative to mandatory legislated standards and can be based on self-assessment or benchmarking. (Benchmarking is something we cover in later chapters.) Best practices are a way for clinicians to standardize clinical practices and business procedures without the oversight of a government agency or state board. Best practices, as you will learn, do require clinicians to collect data and look for ways to continuously improve processes.

---

likely that you will create better, more consistent outcomes. Let us dive deeply into the six patient interaction stations shown in Figure 1–1 by looking at some best practices to be completed at each interaction station.

THE MEMORABLE PATIENT EXPERIENCE

Audiologists must find ways to differentiate their offerings from over-the-counter products and other low-end competitors. One way to do this is by creating a captivating and emotionally engaging patient experience. Design and implementation of the patient experience is the cornerstone of quality. We cover quality as it applies to the clinical process more extensively in later chapters. For now, let us focus on the audiologist's role in the emerging experience-based economy, as it is a great example of how we must broaden our perspective of quality in audiology. No longer is it enough to focus on the all important technical aspects of audiology. We must strive to understand the role audiology services provide in a broader context. That understanding begins by embracing quality from a broad consumer-centric perspective. Design, implementation, and measurement of a memorable patient experience are the path to sustaining quality in a clinical practice.

Since quality is a customer-centric concept, it is best delivered through a remarkable patient experience. In their landmark book, *The Experience Economy*, Pine and Gilmore discuss the use of "best principles." A best principle is a way to create and deliver a customized experience. In contrast to "best practices," which are important for ensuring that diagnostic tests and fitting procedures are accurate, a "best principle" is a way to ensure that you are delivering an authentic, emotionally engaging experience that cannot be duplicated by others. Whereas best practices are procedures that can be copied, a best principle is completely unique to your practice. Pine and Gilmore (2011) discuss using a theme, signature moments and memorabilia to create your customized patient experience. Although none of these concepts are directly related to clinical audiology, all of them are integral to quality; therefore, they are essential to how we practice audiology today.

A theme is a dominant idea or organizing principle that is interwoven through all stages of the patient's interaction with your practice. According to Pine and Gilmore, every practice has a theme. Whether intentional or not, your theme will emerge in the mind of each patient. Sadly, most themes in the audiology world are rather sterile and predictable (like the vast majority of other health care professions). The real opportunity for audiology practices is to find their own theme upon which to build. The general rule for creating a theme for your practice is to make sure it is something that will be emotionally appealing and uplifting to many patients as well as interesting for you and your staff. Some examples of effective themes come from old movies, 1950s cars, and music.

A signature moment is perhaps best described as that breakthrough "A-ha" point in time when you and the patient have established an everlasting bond. The process of selecting and fitting hearing aids on individuals who have suffered from hearing loss for several years is rife with possible signature moments.

They are usually those occasions when the patient has placed their trust in your ability to transform their ability to communicate. Audiologists can use signature moments to build value into their offerings.

Once you have established a theme and signature moment, you can use memorabilia to make the theme or signature moment remarkable to patients. Memorabilia is something that patients can take home as a way to fondly remember the clinical experience. It can be as simple as a colorful, professionally produced brochure. Others may want to go a more exotic route. For example, suppose your theme is 1950s automobiles. You could have miniature '57 Chevys in your reception area and even use engine noise as part of the hearing aid fitting process. Identifying a theme and using memorabilia form the backbone of the six interaction stations comprising the patient experience in an audiology practice, which we examine next.

PROMOTION

Let us consider the waning effectiveness of traditional marketing tactics, such as newspaper ads and direct mail. Once a staple of many practices, we can no longer rely on a consistent pull of new prospects from these traditional marketing media. Given these demographic and socioeconomic constraints, hearing aid dispensing practices must redefine their marketing plans with modern tactics that are designed to build loyalty and create community. In short, the era of plucking low-hanging fruit (hearing aid sales) from a relatively small, captive audience (hearing-impaired patients with no other options to receive hearing care) is over.

Given the rise in electronic media and the evolution in consumer buying habits, the so-called marketing funnel has limited effectiveness. Edelman (2010) has coined the term "loyalty loop" to describe how consumers typically interact with businesses. Rather than attempting to raise awareness of a broad group of prospects and convert a small percentage into sales, the loyalty loop (Figure 1–2) suggests that customers evaluate their options over a longer period of time. Moreover, once they have made a

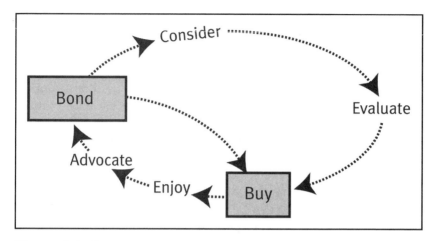

Figure 1–2. The loyalty loop is shown. (Adapted from Edelman, 2010)

buying decision, purchasers want to engage a business in relationship. In contrast to the traditional marketing funnel, which suggests that the buying transaction is the end of the process, the loyalty loop implies that there are opportunities to turn a customer into an advocate or promoter of your business long after the purchase has been made. Data from Edelman (2010) indicate that relationship marketing and electronic media would be two pillars of a modern marketing strategy.

In addition to creating a marketing plan that reaches out to both new and existing patients, there are five distinct marketing tactics that every practice can execute on a monthly basis. We fondly refer to these five tactics as the CORUS of essentials marketing services. Although the core fundamentals of an effective marketing plan are unchanged (e.g., presence in the five pathways, tracking region of interest, a specific allocation of resources devoted to marketing), modernization of your marketing efforts requires a CORUS of new and emerging services. Here is a summary of these CORUS services:

C: Captivating Web site. It is no longer enough to simply have a Web site. Your practice's Web site must have patient-testimonial videos, downloadable educational content, and other interactive material that captivates your prospects and current patients. Perhaps the most important element of a captivating website is an introductory video that addresses the vision and mission of your practice. Rather than showcasing products or technology, this introductory video must speak to the quality-of-life changes hearing aids bring to patients.

O: Online reputation manager. Your Web site also must link current patients to your Web site in order to generate more word-of-mouth referrals. This can be done through an online reputation service, which collects patient testimonials and posts them on your Web site for prospects to view. You can think of an online reputation manager as an electronic version of the traditional pencil-and-paper patient comment card.

R: Relationship and medical marketing programs. Building essential referral networks with physicians and other influencers is no longer a luxury. Physician marketing programs have been available for decades, but many of them fail because the audiologist does not methodically execute the program over a long period of time. Today, building relationships for physicians and other influencers requires that audiologists have a good understanding of comorbidity and disease-state marketing. When hearing care professionals take the time to educate physicians about various disease states, such as diabetes and dementia, and their relationship to hearing loss, it obligates the physician to refer patients to your clinic for a hearing screening.

U: Upstanding member of your community through public relations (PR). Like relationship marketing efforts, PR requires the hearing care professional to have a presence in the community. There are several relevant topics with broad consumer appeal that could be used as part of a systematic PR campaign in your community. Once you have identified a topic that you are passion about and has broad appeal, you can begin to build a PR campaign. Taking a few hours each month to conduct community outreach centered on the installation and use of loop systems is one example of a PR tactic that can brand your practice as a pillar of your community.

S: Social media. Data suggest that more and more people over the age of 70 years are using Facebook and other forms of social media to stay in touch with family and friends. Social media are electronic billboards that allow you to cost-effectively reach an expansive number of current patients and prospects. The key to successful use of social media is your ability to seed your Facebook and Twitter feeds with fresh and informative content that keeps people interested and engaged in your practice.

#DISCOVER

Market Segmentation

In order to manage your marketing budget more efficiently, it is important to conduct some type of segmentation analysis. The purpose of market segmentation is to identify a group of potential customers for your business. Market segmentation takes into consideration the demographics, psychographics, and purchasing behavior of individuals who might be in need of your services. A good market segmentation analysis allows you to pinpoint a specific segment of the market to which you want to market. While answering the question, "What do you want to be known for?" the next step is to find a "market segmentation specialist" in your area that will conduct a market segmentation analysis.

TRADITIONAL MARKETING TACTICS: "GETTING THE BANDD BACK TOGETHER"

BANDD is another acronym used to described promotional tactics clinicians and managers can use in their practice. Of course, the BANDD cannot be outdone by the CORUS. In order to complete our concert of marketing services, there are four traditional marketing tactics that are essential to any comprehensive marketing portfolio. BANDD is the acronym that describes them, and like classic rock, traditional marketing tactics never go out of style. Tapping into your existing database of patients is similar to tapping into your collection of Rolling Stones and The Who —every month or two, you have the urge to listen to something familiar. With database marketing you are tapping into some familiar faces using some of the tactics described below:

B: Brand palette and advertising. A cornerstone of any effective marketing campaign requires a business to have a consistent look and feel to its message. In practical terms, a brand palette is the color, font, logo, tag line, and any other component of how your brand is communicated to the public in its advertising. Once you have established your brand palette you can use it in all your marketing tactics.

A: Advertorials. A variation of public relations is careful placement of advertorials in local newspapers. An advertorial is a short fact-based article of consumer interest that also subtly promotes your practice. There are several topics of interest, such as tinnitus, the dangers of over-the-counter hearing aids, and hearing loops that could be used as subjects in a consumer-oriented advertorial. Many communities have local newspapers and senior newsletters that are willing to features advertorials.

N: Newsletters. Modern printing techniques allow practices to customize their own educational newsletters. Using an office management system, newsletters can be created and mailed to a targeted subsegment of your patient database. Subsegments of your database may include Tested Not Sold, Mild Hearing Loss, and CIC Users.

D: Database letters. Like newsletters, traditional letters with a strong call to action can be sent to specific subsegments of your existing database. Letters to your database can be easily customized using many current office management systems.

D: Digital signage. An emerging technology that warrants further attention for any audiologist interested in modernizing the reception area is Direct Out of Home Marketing.

Direct Out of Home Marketing (DOOH), sometimes called digital signage, has become a very popular educational and advertising delivery vehicle for public and private venues such as retail stores, doctors' offices, and corporate buildings. Recent surveys indicate that DOOH is a useful tool for driving office traffic and consumer buying decisions. In addition to contributing to a modern-looking clinic, there may be some business reasons surrounding the use of DOOH. Cotterill (2011) conducted a digital signage study comparing DOOH with more traditional forms of out of home marketing. Results of this survey showed that "digital signage displays have a 47.7% effectiveness on brand awareness, increased the average purchase amount by 29.5%, created a 31.8% upswing in overall sales volumes and generated a 32.8% growth in repeat buyers." According to Dodson (2011) the core to DOOH marketing is the use of digital signage, which is displayed in the reception area on a flat screen television. The content of the digital signage displayed on the flat screen television is usually controlled using basic personal computers, by way of proprietary software programs. This keeps the costs of DOOH manageable by avoiding any large capital outlays for the controller equipment. Most systems automatically update themselves using a high-speed Internet connection, which reduces clinic staff involvement and keeps fresh content in front of your patients. The hearing care professional simply has to inform the DOOH service of changes and updates in content that is displayed on the flat screen television.

PHONE SCHEDULING

The next interaction station common to all audiology practices is phone scheduling. The act of answering the phone, answering questions, and booking appointments are all components of this interaction station. The essential behavioral underpinnings of phone scheduling is a friendly voice, the ability to concisely answer questions posed by patients, and to schedule appointments. The metrics used to measure phone scheduling are number of calls received and the number of appointments booked per day. Chapter 4 is mainly devoted to the quality surrounding this all important interaction station.

@CONNECT

In addition to being process oriented, quality is patient centered. The proof that a procedure, test, or best practice is effective is if it results in a more satisfied patient or a better outcome; thus, the gathering of various dimensions of outcome forms the underpinnings of quality. This is called "voice of customer" information in quality-control parlance. For more information, follow @CustomersFocus on Twitter.

ARRIVAL

Design of the patient experience requires the hearing care professional to "theme" their practice. Using memorabilia that is interesting to a broad segment of your target audience, you can choose a theme revolving around something about which you are passionate. Classic cars, movie musicals, and pets are some examples of popular themes.

If you are familiar with Disney World's business model, you might know something about the concept of "theming." Theming in a hearing aid dispensing or audiology practice usually begins with design of a more appealing waiting room. We are all familiar with the adage that you never get a second chance to make a good first impression. That certainly holds true for the patient's arrival in your waiting area. Using the five senses, hearing care professionals are encouraged to turn the waiting room into an event, rather than drudgery (Mahdavi, 2011). An inviting reception area and a friendly greeting by office staff are the pillars of the arrival interaction station.

TESTING AND RECOMMENDATION

Regardless of the lifestyle, budget constraints, age, or hearing loss of the individual adult patient, there are four vital pieces of information that need to be gathered during prefitting assessment conducted on every adult patient:

1. Buying priorities of the patient (price, cosmetics, performance, ease of use)
2. Self-perception of the communication problem and readiness for help
3. Communication ability in everyday listening situations
4. Extent of the hearing/communication deficit.

Each of these components can be obtained using traditional means; however, to differentiate one's practice from the competition, an audiologist must identify ways to emotionally connect with his or her patient and engage them in an otherwise sterile and ordinary clinical process. Let us examine each of these four components and review tools and procedures allowing audiologists to bring each to life for their patients.

BUYING PRIORITIES OF THE PATIENT

According to Baker (1995) the typical customer makes a buying decision based on one of four priorities: (1) cosmetics ("I like the way it looks"); (2) performance ("I like the way it works"); (3) ease of use/flexibility ("I like how simple it is to use"); or (4) price ("I got a good deal"). During the prefitting assessment it is important to identify which of those four dimensions is the highest priority for each patient. The buying preference matrix can be used to classify what the most important buying priority might be for each patient. The buying preference matrix is not a form or questionnaire; rather, it is a method used to classify observable patient behavior gathered during the early stages of the prefitting assessment (Figure 1–3). As you would expect, patients often do not fit completely into just one quad-

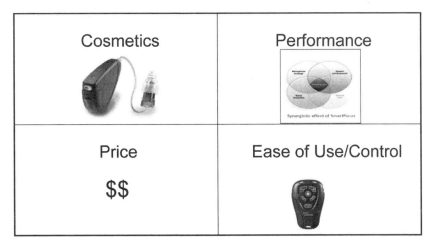

Figure 1–3. The buying-preference matrix is shown.

rant; rather, they often have a high priority and a second priority. The main point of using the buying preference matrix approach is to allow the practitioner to reframe how hearing-impaired patients approach the market for his or her services and then tailor your message in a way that resonates with the patient. Using the four-quadrant buying preference matrix to classify the priorities of the individual patient has a secondary effect. Given the abundance of features found on today's hearing aids, it is critical that you do not overwhelm the patient with too much information. Classifying the patient's buying preferences using this matrix helps avoid the problem of "burying the lead," which is a phrase used to describe providing your patients with too much information.

Another way to streamline the gathering of patient information during the prefitting assessment is the prudent use of questionnaires. Questionnaires are a tool that helps you gather information from the patient in a more formal manner. Questionnaires that patients complete in the reception area prior to their appointment allow you to have a more focused conversation with the patient. In addition to the four-quadrant buying preference matrix, questionnaires can be used to gather additional information. According to Poost-Foroosh, Jennings, and Cheesman (2012) questionnaires, such as the Hearing Handicap

Inventory for the Elderly (HHIE; Ventry & Weinstein, 1982) can be used to better understand the individual needs of the patient and form the foundation for patient-centric care, which is an important component of quality.

Using a questionnaire, such as the Characteristics of Amplification Tool (COAT) created by Sandridge and Newman (2006), allows the audiologist to efficiently quantify many hearing aid selection issues, including buying preferences. The COAT can be administered to the patient prior to the appointment. The information gathered on the COAT allows the professional to tailor the prefitting appointment to better meet the needs of the individual by asking questions about style preference and priorities with regard to new product usage.

READINESS FOR HELP

There is little correlation between objective audiological test results and a patient's readiness to pursue amplification (see Taylor, 2007, for a review). On the other hand, a patient's willingness to accept help and use hearing aids is correlated with the patient's self-perceived hearing handicap (Laplante-Levesque, Hickson, & Worrall, 2012). Over the years, questionnaires have been developed to quantify self-perception of hearing handicap. The Hearing Handicap Inventory for the Elderly (HHIE) developed by Ventry and Weinstein (1982) and the Hearing Performance Inventory (HPI) developed by Hawes and Niswander (1985) are two more commonly mentioned questionnaires in the literature. Although these questionnaires and others like them have been scientifically validated, they are not widely used clinically. Some of the reasons for their lack of popularity may include that they are difficult to score and administer or too time-consuming and cumbersome for patients to complete.

Palmer, Solodar, Hurley, Byrne, and Williams (2009) evaluated the use of a single question as a determinant of patient readiness for amplification. That question was, "On a scale of 1 to 10, 1 being the worst and 10 being the best, how would you rate your overall hearing ability?" Results of their study indicated that the study participants' responses to this question were repeatable; thus, the authors concluded that the answer to this question provided by a patient during an actual appointment was reliable and valid. Given the findings from this study, hearing care professionals could systematically ask and record the answer to this question during the prefitting assessment in order to gauge patients' perception of a hearing handicap as well as their readiness for amplification.

COMMUNICATION ABILITY IN EVERYDAY LISTENING SITUATIONS

Your ability to ask thought-provoking, open-ended questions and listen to understand usually leads to an in-depth dialogue with the patient about communication ability in everyday listening situations. From a consultative perspective, the purpose of asking these questions during the prefitting assessment is to target a specific list of communication priorities for the patient. One tool that has been used successfully is the Client Oriented Scale of Improvement (COSI). The COSI is an open-ended communication assessment and outcome measure tool that allows the patient to nominate up to five areas to target for improvement. The COSI is so popular that many hearing aid manufacturers include it in their software.

Another communication assessment tool is the TELEGRAM (Figure 1–4). The TELEGRAM, created by Thibodeau (2004), is a semi-open-ended communication assessment tool requiring the patient and audiologist to evaluate communication on a 1 to 5 scale across more than 10 specific listening situations. Similar to the COSI, it allows the audiologist to record and target three listening situations unique to the individual. Unlike the COSI, the TELEGRAM also allows the audiologist to record specific recommendations in relation to the listening situations listed on the form. For example, the TELEGRAM allows the audiologist and patient to rate communication ability using a cell phone and landline telephone.

Using the findings of MarkeTrak, you can use the COSI or TELEGRAM to build a case for recommending a customized solution, which usually requires advanced hearing aid technology.

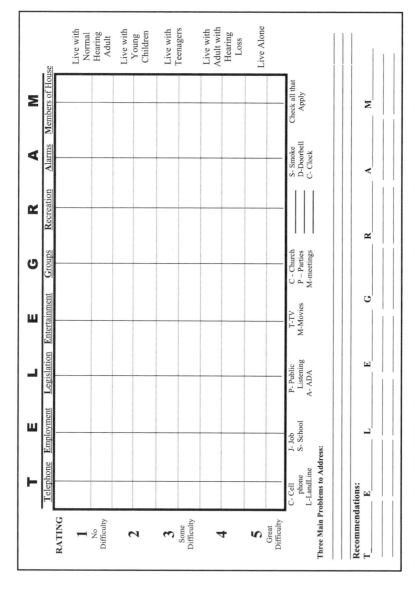

Figure 1–4. The TELEGRAM unaided assessment tool is shown. (Adapted from Thibodeau, 2004)

Multiple Environment Listening Utility (MELU) is a term coined by Sergei Kochkin that describes a patient's ability to benefit from amplification across several different everyday listening situations. MELU is strongly associated with overall satisfaction (Kochkin, 2011). MarkeTrak data suggest that patient satisfaction exceeds 80% when a patient is benefitting from amplification in 10 or more discrete listening situations. This suggests the audiologist and patient could target and rate 10 or more listening situations in the unaided condition during a routine prefitting appointment. Because it allows you to rate 10 or more distinct listening situations, the TELEGRAM is a useful tool for accomplishing this task and can be completed *before* the audiologic test battery is administered.

EXTENT OF THE COMMUNICATION DEFICIT

Once a medical pathology has been ruled out, the primary purpose of the auditory test battery is to quantify the residual auditory capacity and determine hearing aid candidacy of the individual. The efficacy of various procedures used to complete these tasks has been well documented. For example, loudness discomfort level (LDL) measures should be routinely conducted in order to program the hearing aid's maximum power output (Mueller, 2011). Many of the required auditory tests are mandated by individual state licensing laws; however, whenever possible, hearing care professionals should identify areas of the test battery that can be modernized with the intent of providing a more meaningful experience for the patient. Given the number of patient complaints associated with speech understanding in background noise, a logical target for modernization is speech audiometry. For several reasons, speech-in-noise testing must be incorporated into the prefitting hearing aid assessment. Firstly, it measures the primary complaint of most patients, which is an inability to understand speech in the presence of background noise. Secondly, patients routinely comment that, unlike puretone audiometry or speech testing in quiet using single words, speech-in-noise testing is actually measuring the problem that brought them to the clinic. Thirdly, speech-in-noise test scores can be easily used in the counseling and recommendation phases of the prefitting assessments. There is also strong evidence supporting the efficacy of speech-in-noise testing when both single words and sentence-length stimuli are utilized. Killion, Niquette, Gudmundsen, Revit, and Banerjee, et al. (2004) showed that the Quick Speech-in-Noise (Quick SIN) test can be reliably used to assess signal-to-noise (SNR) loss in adults. Wilson (2011) used the Words-in-Noise (WIN) test to compare word recognition in quiet to word recognition in noise performance for a group of 3,430 veterans. His results showed that of the over 3,000 veterans tested with abnormal performance on the WIN, almost half (46%) had excellent performance on word recognition in quiet, and 21.5% with abnormal performance on the WIN test had good word recognition in quiet performance. Wilson concluded that listening in quiet and listening in noise are two different domains of auditory function; thus, both should be routinely assessed. It is the responsibility of the audiologist to select a validated sentence-length or single-word test that uses noise to "stress" the auditory system during the prefitting assessment. Among the best choices would be either the Quick SIN or WIN test.

Although similar to word recognition ability, annoyance from noise is a separate domain of auditory function worthy of assessment during the prefitting appointment. In a series of well-publicized studies from the University of Tennessee (e.g., Nabelek, Freyaldenhoven, Tampas, & Burchfield, 2006) using the Acceptable Noise Level (ANL) test, it has been documented that annoyance from noise levels may be a predictor of hearing aid use rates. Given this evidence, combined with the fact that the ANL test has reasonable face validity; it should also be a routine part of the prefitting assessment.

The well-respected audiologist, Robert Sweetow, has proposed the use of a "functional communication assessment," in which two objective and two subjective measures of the residual auditory system are used. For these reasons routine testing of speech intelligibility in noise and annoyance from sound would be warranted prior to prescribing amplification. The Red Flag Matrix has been put forth by Taylor and Bernstein (2011) as a practical method for documenting the results of two speech-in-noise tests that measure two different domains of the auditory system. It provides a way to more clearly articulate the results of two speech-in-noise tests in a more meaningful way to patients.

As disruptive innovations and consumer buying behavior evolve, hearing care professionals must keep pace. These changes in the marketplace necessitate not only the use of evidence-based test protocols but clinical procedures that engage and captivate the patient. The four prefitting procedures in this article are designed to create a more memorable patient experience. By delivering this experience, using the best clinical evidence to support their implementation is a proven approach for differentiating your practice from low-cost retailers and over-the-counter PSAPS. Through the combination of scientific evidence-based application of clinical research and the judicious use of "high touch" service, audiologists are poised to meet the demands on the new consumer in the uncertain economy. Let us briefly review the final two interaction stations. Chapter 3 goes into considerably more detail on quality surrounding patient benefit and satisfaction.

FITTING AND PURCHASE

Once the appropriate amplification device has been selected, the patient goes through a step-by-step fitting process. This process requires the audiologist to orientate and instruct the patient about proper care, use, and expectation surrounding initial use of the devices. Verification of performance is completed using probe-microphone measures. At the end of the fitting appointment, the patient usually makes the purchase by paying with a credit card. Chapter 3 goes into the details of best practices for fitting and purchase.

FOLLOW-UP

A series of appointments are made during the follow-up phase of the patient journey. Included in these appointments would be validation of the hearing aid fitting using self-reports of real-world benefit. Also included in the follow-up appointment would be auditory training, personal adjustment counseling, fine-tuning of the instruments, and troubleshooting. Chapter 3 provides more details on issues related to quality during the follow-up phase of the patient journey.

@*CONNECT*

Kraig Kramers

Kramers is the author of CEO Tools. He often talks about the methodical nature of management. For us, we can think of quality as one component of vigilant management. This includes the ability to hire the right people, set proper expectations, and align strategy with tactics in order to run your practice. Even though a comprehensive practice modernization program is needed to overcome the demands of the ever changing market, effective implementation requires old-fashioned management vigilance. There are seven actions in which all effective managers must engage with their staff in order to implement a clinic modernization program. When you get right down to it, however, the action required to move a business ahead needs to come from the manager. The essence of effective management is summarized in Figure 1–5. Those are the seven actions needed to move any new initiative ahead in an organization, including those related to quality. The key words are focus and action. Without taking some type of action, your business is doomed to fail, and without the proper focus, your actions will be wasted. It is up to the manager to decide which actions take priority. Following the steps on the wheel will help you focus and take action. There is really no special or unique talent to run a good business or to be a good manager—just the ability to do the right things.

Now that we have choreographed the six interaction stations of the patient experience, we can begin the process of learning

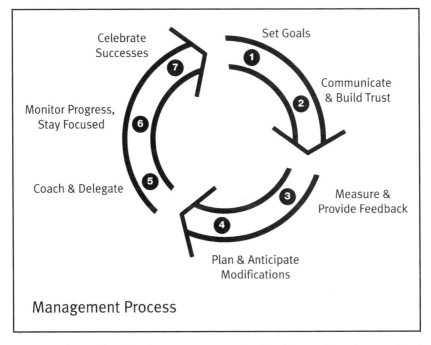

Figure 1–5. The 7-point management wheel based on the work of Kraig Kramers of CEO Tools, Inc.

more about the conceptual foundation of quality. The rest of this chapter tackles the concept of quality as it is broadly defined.

Historically, productivity was the most important dimension of business performance. Success was largely defined by how many widgets a factory could produce each day, not by the quality of the widgets. The most successful businesses were those that could more efficiently outproduce their competitors. In other words, the more widgets your factory made, the more likely they were to beat the competition and gain a larger share of the consumer's wallet. Throughout the twentieth century, this economic model, which was an outgrowth of the industrial revolution, held true for most businesses, including health care. For health care practices, a business model based on productivity meant that physicians billed based on the number of tests and procedures they ordered, not on the outcome of their treatment decisions. For hearing aid dispensing practices, which are a derivative of the health care business model, this meant that professionals were paid based on the number of "sales" rather than the final outcome of their fittings. Figure 1–6 describes the three fundamental drivers of the hearing aid practices.

As technology has improved and costs have been reduced, consumers have had more choices and they have demanded more features, lower prices, and better service; thus, productivity alone has become an insufficient gauge of business performance. Although health care has some important differences compared with other businesses, productivity alone is an ineffective way to judge the success of any health care-related business, including hearing aid dispensing. As this book illustrates, audiologists must clearly define, orchestrate, and measure quality in their practices if they are to thrive in the 21st century.

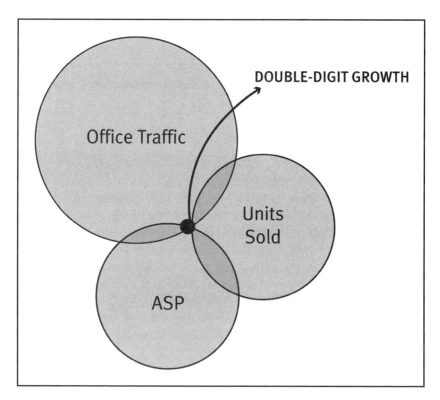

Figure 1–6. Productivity Venn diagram is shown. *ASP*, Average Selling Price.

#*DISCOVER*

Frederick Winslow Taylor (1856–1915)

Taylor is regarded as the father of scientific management and industrial efficiency. Many of his theories led to the creation of a "top-down" management hierarchy in which professional managers broke down assembly line tasks into incremental segments. His early 20th century innovations in factory labor workflow led to breakthroughs in business efficiency.

Taylor's scientific management consisted of four principles:

1. Replace rule-of-thumb work methods with methods based on a scientific study of the tasks.
2. Scientifically select, train, and develop each employee rather than passively leaving them to train themselves.
3. Provide detailed instruction and supervision of each worker in the performance of that worker's discrete task.
4. Divide work nearly equally between managers and workers, so that the managers apply scientific management principles to planning the work and the workers actually perform the tasks.

Although many of Taylor's innovations are thought of as draconian in nature by today's standards, his influence lives on. If you have ever had a factory job that required you to punch the time clock or go through a rigorous on-the-job training program, you have encountered a century-old "Taylorism."

THE FOUNDATIONS OF QUALITY

Since the term "quality" is an abstract concept, it is important that we spend some time addressing what this term means. Let us begin by comparing the concept of "quality" with the similar concept of "excellence." All clinicians have the desire to take care of their patients. After all, that is why many people get into so-called helping professions, such as audiology; however, just having the desire to be a great caregiver does not mean you have a high-quality practice. Possessing the desire to provide outstanding patient care and delivering a high-quality outcome to patients is really the difference between excellence and quality. These are two concepts that are intimately related, yet different. Although the concepts are similar, there are some important differences that need to be addressed.

If you are a football fan, you may have heard legendary football coaches, such as Paul "Bear" Bryant and Vince Lombardi, talk about a "commitment to excellence." Perhaps you are wondering why they emphasized excellence, rather than quality, in their pep talks to their teams. Even though they were addressing their teams, they knew teams are composed of a group of individuals. In order to win, they knew each of the individuals had to play their best. Excellence is an intrinsic construct that can be defined as an individual's ability to provide their best effort and continually try to improve. It is our innate desire to go above and beyond to deliver a superior service experience or outcome. You may hear people refer to the profession as a "calling." Many professionals expect themselves to exceed the expectations of the patient. When we go above the call of duty to help a patient, we are expressing a commitment to excellence.

Quality, on the other hand, is the standardization of excellence. It is an extrinsic construct. It is the collectively individual commitment to excellence that improves the overall quality of an organization. The critical difference between quality and excellence is that quality is defined and driven by external standards. When we implement a best practices standard that is consistent with industry norms, we are using quality to manage our practice. Mapping out a new clinical process, such as the one outlined earlier in this chapter, we are standardizing a commitment to excellence through quality initiatives. When we utilize checklists and other proxy measures, we are standardizing a commitment to excellence through quality control.

The one factor that can distinguish your practice from others is an obsession with quality. Quality is a broadly defined concept that involves, at its core, leadership, innovation, and inspiration. Focusing on quality, in the broadest sense of the term, requires audiologists to look beyond test results, units sold, and hearing aid technology to systematize processes for both patients and employees. To move from an intrinsic commitment to excellence to a business defined by quality requires a foundation built on three ingredients. These three foundational ingredients are culture, process, and results. This is also known as the Quality Trinity. Each core component is shown in Figure 1–7. Let us examine each of these components in more detail.

CULTURE COUNTS

There is no shortage of business management experts touting the importance of leadership in running an organization. Authority figures from former General Electric CEO Jack Welch to Professor Jim Collins, author of the best-selling book *Good to Great*, all emphasize the need for effective leadership throughout any organization. Perhaps the most important role for any leader of a business is to establish the culture of the organization. Like the term quality, "culture" is difficult to define. In essence, culture

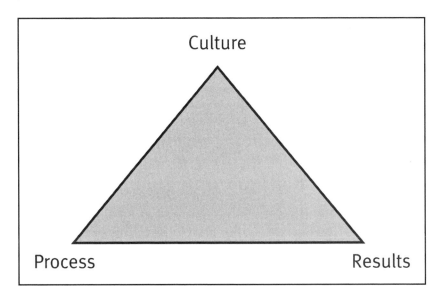

Figure 1–7. The three primary ingredients of quality are shown.

is the acceptable customs, mores, and practices within a group of people. All of us understand culture on a large scale. Shaking someone's hand when we first meet, rather than giving them a hug and kiss, is typically a very acceptable practice in the United States. It is part of American culture. If you hang out at the local pub every Friday night with a group of friends, you might talk about football and hunting, but never politics. That is another example of culture on a very small scale. Even a small audiology practice with a couple of staff has a culture. In a business all the people within the organization, starting with the owner, managers, and leaders, set the tone of your culture.

As you begin to raise the bar on quality within your practice, it is essential to foster a culture based on shared purpose and values. Some practices still subscribe to the outworn management doctrine that leadership is about conveying ideas from the boss' head to the employees' hands. This is the antiquated management principle pioneered by Frederick Taylor more than 100 years ago. Innovative practices, on the other hand, are actively engaged in building management capital through quality. These practices have developed metrics that regularly assess quality. Additionally, these practices that focus on quality foster an environment allowing professionals to act, learn, and make decisions about how to provide superior value to patients.

If you find yourself in a situation in which you are managing a practice, the first priority must be to establish a culture dedicated—maybe even slightly obsessed with—quality. The underpinnings of establishing a culture of quality revolves around four elements: people, inspiration, practice, and environment. This is called the PIPE model of culture building (Mahdavi, 2011). As a person who takes a leadership position within a practice, it is your responsibility to set the stage by emphasizing these four elements.

> **People:** Make sure you hire people that espouse your values. In addition to a commitment to excellence, people need to have the mindset of continuous quality improvement.
>
> **Inspiration:** Use effective communication strategies to ensure you inspire the people you hire. People who feel genuinely inspired will deliver better outcomes to those they serve.

Practice: Inspired people must be given opportunities to practice their skills and freely make mistakes on their career journey of continual self-improvement.

Environment: The physical setting and the mental space of your employees need to be taken into consideration. Make sure you provide an environment that allows your staff to feel nurtured and secure.

Perhaps the most critical element of culture is self-improvement. Rather than focusing on being good, professionals who promote quality must focus on getting better. Fostering a culture based on incremental self-improvement, rather than being good, is thought to make individuals more successful in their careers (Grant-Halvorson, 2012). A culture dedicated to continuous self-improvement is an essential underpinning of quality.

@*CONNECT*

Bill George

George is the former CEO of Medtronic and author of the book *True North*. He is also a professor at the Harvard School of Business. For insights on culture, leadership, and quality follow him on Twitter @BillGeorge.

PROCESS MATTERS

Another foundational ingredient of quality is the consistent use of processes and protocols to manage your business. You can think of process as the step-by-step workflow of your business. The use of disciplined and consistent processes is an essential aspect of quality. Although processes need to be regimented, they also need to have some flexibility. Some quality experts use the term "process thinking." This means that the manager must know what "inputs" or activities are required in order to achieve a desired output. Once these activities are known, the manager of quality must be able to orchestrate a sequence of events that culminate in a superior result (Gupta, 2007). In reality, process thinking necessitates that some audiologists change their mindsets. Rather than focusing on the number of tests and hearing aids fitted, the quality of the outcome for each individual needs to be emphasized. The tools, metrics, and processes discussed throughout this book, when executed properly, should result in higher quality patient outcomes.

PATIENT-CENTRIC RESULTS

In the past, results or outcomes were determined by the professional, not the customer or patient. Partly as a result of the quality movement in other sectors of the economy, heath care systems are evolving that are consumer driven. In this consumer-driven model, it is the patient, not the practitioner, who chiefly decides on the final outcome of any treatment or recommendation. In this consumer-centric era, the major indexes of quality are real-world results. As you will learn, a primary method of measuring real-world results is the use of questionnaires, which capture the patient's impression of your treatment recommendations.

Let us use hearing aid fitting results as an example. The way you would monitor and improve the results of your fittings would be to first establish a process for how you would conduct a fitting appointment. All tests and procedures would be itemized in your process. The next step would be to develop a system of key performance indicators, including a system for collecting the data. Finally, you would designate a person on your staff to monitor the data relative to hearing aid fitting outcomes. This is a very methodical process that very few audiologists routinely perform.

LEARNING FROM MANUFACTURERS

Hearing aid manufacturers have relied on a system of standardized processes designed to improve quality for several years. At the heart of these standardized processes is a desire to reduce variance in their products and processes. In other words, it does matter if you order the hearing aid from Manufacturer X's lab in Canada or Manufacturer X's lab in Europe, because both audiologists (and ultimately each patient) will be receiving devices that meet the same set of performance standards. This reliance on a predetermined set of standards and the underlying manufacturing processes used to make hearing aids did not get created out of a vacuum. There is actually a rich history of "quality control" worth exploring in some detail. It should not come as too much of a surprise, given the automobile's universal importance to modern life, that the automobile industry has popularized many facets of the quality control movement over the past 75 years. Given the market demand for a safe and reliable car, automobile manufacturers were forced to embrace quality initiatives several decades ago. Because Japanese auto makers were the first to implement quality initiatives, they enjoyed a significant advantage in terms of both customer satisfaction and profitability as compared with their American competitions, who have only recently begun to close the quality gap.

Due to international competitive pressures after World War II, American manufacturers were forced to embrace quality management techniques in order to improve business performance. Over several decades, quality management techniques have evolved to meet this challenge. The essential concept underlying each of these quality management techniques is that they are data-driven approaches to improving business results. In order to gain a more thorough understanding of how quality can be managed, let us review some of the most significant quality management techniques used by manufacturers.

Starting in the 1970s, Japanese auto makers challenged the supremacy of the United States' car industry. A significant part of Japan's rise in the auto industry rested on their ability to use data to improve manufacturing processes. Even though they lost their dominance in the 1970s and 1980s, these lessons were not lost on American manufacturers, as several quality management techniques pioneered in Japan were introduced around the world throughout this period. Although many of these quality management techniques were brought to the United States from Japan in the late 1970s and early 1980s, it was not until the 1990s that they were widely embraced by American auto companies.

@CONNECT

Data-Driven Decision Making

The concept of "data-driven decision making" might be new to some people. A good way to think about how "data-driven" decisions are used in a business comes from the book (and subsequent movie) *Moneyball*. Rather than relying on intuition and instinct, which are known to often lead to biased decisions, the general manager of the Oakland Athletics used certain key performance indicators (KPIs) to make personnel decisions. *Moneyball* is a treatise on how dispassionate, data-driven decisions trump experience and intuition in the world of professional baseball. You don't need to know anything about America's pastime to appreciate the data-driven decision-making process. Many of the upcoming chapters go into considerable detail on KPIs and data-driven decisions, but for now you might want to connect with Quality Management Tools to learn more about data-driven decision-making processes. Go to @Quality_ Management on Twitter.

The length of time it took these techniques to become adapted in the face of eroding market share from their Japanese competitors over the 20-year period speaks to the importance of company culture. It was not until companies made the decision to allow these quality techniques to permeate their entire organization that they began to regain lost market share.

Another example of the data-driven decision-making process rests with performance control charts. Performance control charts are a method of logging information about the critical tasks and key outcomes of the manufacturing process. Performance control charts bring together the disciplines of statistics, engineering, and economics to improve the consistency of production processes. In the 1980s more elaborate data-driven systems that led to higher quality outcomes in manufacturing were introduced. This list includes International Organization for Standardization (ISO) 9000, Baldridge Criteria for Business Excellence, and Jiran's Quality Trilogy. These early quality management techniques led to improved business performance, which in turn led to an increase in consumer expectations and demand for products that were better, faster, and cheaper. The spiral of demand and supply changed the paradigm from a focus on quantity to a focus on quality. In order to meet the rising expectations of consumers, quality management systems had to evolve.

Most of us may recall from a statistics course that the Greek letter sigma is used to represent the standard deviation of a data set. Of course, the more deviation from the norm (a big sigma, so to speak), the more that particular data point varies. A systematic reduction in variation in any process is really the essence of something called Six Sigma. In the 1980s, Motorola, which was facing unprecedented competitive pressures in the electronics industry, developed Six Sigma. Using benchmarking data, customer feedback, and systematic analysis, the Six Sigma process was originally designed to reduce variance in the manufacturing process. Six Sigma is a process in which no more than 3.4 defects per million opportunities/chances can occur.

Six Sigma is a methodology for improving performance. The essence of Six Sigma requires that each step in the manufacturing process use data to reduce defects. Over the past two decades Six Sigma itself has evolved into a highly complex quality management system; however, the essence of Six Sigma is using voice-of-customer (VOC) data to develop key business indicators and process maps. As you will read throughout this book, those critical underpinnings of Six Sigma can be applied to practice management and hearing aid dispensing. Now is a good time to look back to Figure 1–1. The six interaction stations are a simple example of the Six Sigma "value stream." A value stream is a sequence of process steps that convert materials, services, and information into a sellable product in which customers see value. The fundamental goal of Six Sigma is to create value for customers while achieving business objectives through the reduction in process variance. You might be thinking that Six Sigma works well for making products, such as hearing aids, but does any of it really apply to running an audiology practice? Believe it or not, certain concepts of Six Sigma, namely VOC data collection and value-stream analysis can be implemented into your practice if you are dedicated to improving the quality of care and patient outcomes.

@*CONNECT*

Voice of Customer and Six Sigma

An integral part of Six Sigma is collecting and analyzing information for customers. Voice of customer (VOC) is actually an in-depth technique for capturing customer data that can be used to make decisions about quality. Much has been written about this process, and there are many possible ways to gather the information (focus groups, individual interviews, contextual inquiry, ethnographic techniques, etc.), but all involve a series of structured in-depth interviews which focus on customers' experiences with current products or alternatives within the category under consideration. Needs statements are then extracted, organized into a more usable hierarchy, and then prioritized by customers. To learn more about VOC in the Six Sigma process visit @iSixSigma on Twitter.

One of the most current iterations of Six Sigma involves something commonly known by a five-letter acronym, DMAIC. DMAIC is a five-step data-driven quality improvement approach that stands for define, measure, analyze, improve, and control. DMAIC, which is summarized in Figure 1–8, is a disciplined quality management approach that uses data for making informed decisions about your organization.

Since DMAIC has several applications to the practice of audiology, let us examine each of the five steps more carefully:

1. Define—The define phase establishes the objective for improving the processes, methods, and standards. This is a well-defined and clear step in which VOC data, process analysis, and overall quality assessment data are used. The gaps in quality between the actual and target performance are identified.
2. Measure—The measure phase starts with understanding the assumptions, problems, and challenges associated with collecting data around a clearly defined objective. Data are collected that can be compared with a predefined benchmark.

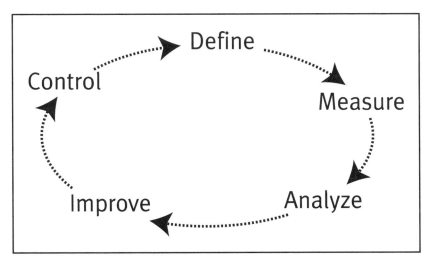

Figure 1–8. The DMAIC components.

3. Analyze—The analyze phase requires that you examine the data you collected looking for causes of quality problems, costs associated with those problems, and detailed brainstorming around possible solutions.
4. Improve—During this phase you enact action plans around possible solutions you have determined. Included in this phase are all financial and organizational issues related to the solutions listed.
5. Control—Using data to fine-tune and continuously improve around the objectives listed in the first step of DMAIC.

Hearing aid manufacturers have relied on many of the quality techniques outlined above for more than 30 years in an effort to incrementally improve the quality and reliability of their devices. Hearing aid manufacturers typically use the return rate as one key performance indicator. Manufacturers use a combination of objective and subjective measures to incrementally reduce variation in products and improve quality. For example, hearing aid manufacturers use long-term (45 days) and short-term (15 days) returns for credit data to make decisions about quality process improvements and product defects. Using Pareto's 80/20 rule, the quality team at the manufacturer looks for potential trends in the data that would indicate a "red flag" for a product defect.

@CONNECT

W. Edwards Deming (1900–1993)

Responsible for pioneering the Total Quality Movement, Deming was originally shunned by American manufacturing moguls, so he went to Japan where he pioneered his 14-point quality system. Although it may seem obvious now, Deming was the first to believe that manufacturing was really a system of interwoven events, rather than silos of experts. Deming was also responsible for fostering the concept of continuous improvement in the manufacturing process. Here is a summary of Deming's 14 points:

1. Create constancy of purpose toward improvement of product and service, with the aim to become competitive, stay in business, and provide jobs.
2. Adopt the new philosophy. We are in a new economic age. Western management must awaken to the challenge, learn their responsibilities, and take on leadership for change.
3. Cease dependence on inspection to achieve quality. Eliminate the need for massive inspection by building quality into the product in the first place.
4. End the practice of awarding business on the basis of a price tag; instead, minimize total cost. Move toward a single supplier for any one item, in a long-term relationship of loyalty and trust.
5. Improve constantly and forever the system of production and service, to improve quality and productivity, and thus constantly decrease costs.
6. Institute training on the job.
7. Institute leadership. The aim of supervision should be to help people as well as machines and gadgets do a better job.
8. Drive out fear, so that everyone can work effectively for the company.

9. Break down barriers between departments. People in research, design, sales, and production must work as a team in order to foresee problems of production and usage that may be encountered with the product or service.
10. Eliminate slogans, exhortations, and targets for the work force asking for zero defects and new levels of productivity.
11. a. Eliminate work quotas on the factory floor; instead, substitute with leadership.
    b. Eliminate management by objective. Eliminate management by numbers and numerical goals; instead substitute with leadership.
12. a. Remove barriers that rob the hourly worker of his right to pride of workmanship. The responsibility of supervisors must be changed from sheer numbers to quality.
    b. Remove barriers that rob people in management and engineering of their right to pride of workmanship. This means, *inter alia*, abolishment of the annual or merit rating and of management by objective.
13. Institute a vigorous program of education and self-improvement.
14. Put everybody in the company to work to accomplish the transformation. The transformation is everybody's job.

(The 80/20 rule implies that the quality team is looking for consistent patterns or trends in the reasons for returns, i.e., 80% of the problem is caused by 20% of the possibilities.) If a trend in the data suggests there is a product or component defect, the quality team performs something called a root-cause analysis to identify the core reason for the defect. Most audiologists are not too familiar with the term "root cause analysis." Although quality experts in manufacturing have created all sorts of elaborate mechanisms for conducting a root cause analysis (e.g., "Fishboning") the underlying core concept of a root cause analysis is brainstorming with your team to identify a list of possible causes for defects or variances in outcomes, and then implementing a plan to close the gap in defects or variance after the "root cause" has been isolated. After the root cause of the defect is identified, the quality team establishes a change in process or training that is likely to eliminate or reduce the defect. After adjustments are made in processes, the quality team continues to monitor both objective and subjective data, much of it coming directly from customers. As DMAIC (see Figure 1–8) suggests, quality is a continuous process that relies on a feedback loop to close gaps in variance.

Over time, the quality team uses data to modify or change a manufacturing procedure. The continual collection of data as well as systematic meetings of the team to review data and examine trends, combined with modifications and changes based on the data, results is a cyclical feedback loop which results in continuous incremental improvement.

#DISCOVER

Minitab Statistical Software

Six Sigma and other quality initiatives require that data not only be collected, but that they be analyzed properly before decisions are made. The process of analyzing data in order to find statistical significance can be easily done with software. One example is Minitab, which allows managers of quality a fast and accurate way to know their analysis is statistically significant. Even though you may never have to analyze data in your clinic to this degree of certainly before making a decision, it is good to know it exists. Go to http://www.minitab.com to find this software. Later chapters address how outcome data can be used to fine-tune best practice processes.

Audiologists can learn a considerable amount about quality from their colleagues in manufacturing. Specifically, audiologists can apply the concepts of DMAIC to identify variances in process and defects in products or patient outcomes. For audiologists, the hearing aid fitting and its outcome would be considered the process that is most prone to variance. Various outcome measures (see Chapter 3), which serve as the objective and subjective measures, would be used to identify process gaps and defects. A root-cause analysis could be conducted to identify reasons for these gaps and defects. Once a root cause has been identified, audiologists could develop corrective and preventive actions to reduce or eliminate the defects. This is likely to involve an adjustment to how a procedure or test is conducted by the audiologist in the clinic.

LEARNING FROM HEALTH CARE

Historically, the health care sector of the economy in the U.S. has struggled with quality relative to the manufacturing sector. This statement is supported by the fact that one in four patients are harmed by medical errors, and the wrong person or wrong body part is operated on 40 times per week (Makary, 2012). A significant part of the quality problems associated with health care in the United States is a lack of transparency. Furthermore, physicians have not been accountable for providing outcome data to consumers. In other words, patients do not have access to data, such as infection and complication rates for hospitals, that might help them make decisions about where to go (and places to avoid) for various medical procedures. Also, physicians and other medical staff do not have an incentive to change or improve when their results are not being monitored by consumers.

The lesson for audiologists is that outcome measures (i.e., the results of the fitting) for hearing aid dispensing practices should be transparent to the public. Over the past few years, a growing number of hospitals and clinics have made complication and infection rates available to the public. Not only does this data make informed decisions possible for patients, but it creates an incentive for health care practitioners and physicians to focus on quality of outcomes because they are being judged by consumers of their services. Audiologists would be wise to learn from medical practices that are publicizing their outcomes to the public by developing some type of a scorecard that consumers would be able to evaluate prior to making decisions about where to receive services. Considering audiology services are a hybrid business, delivering transparent information to consumers might be a less painful feat compared with the resistance to transparency by some physicians as outlined by Makary (2012).

According to the Institute of Medicine of the National Academies, the definition of quality for medical professionals is patient care that is safe, effective, efficient, evidence based, patient centered, and timely. This is a good starting point for the dispensing audiologist's definition of quality, but it is incomplete for the following reason: Unlike other medical specialties, hearing aid dispensing is unique in that it is a hybrid business model. Although it is not the only hybrid business model in the allied medical professions (plastic surgery and optometry come to mind) hearing aid dispensing is the merging of both medical and retail professions. From a medical orientation, there is no doubt that audiologists and other hearing health care providers use their training and expertise to treat patients. Any time an audiologist completes a comprehensive auditory assessment or cerumen removal, they are working in the medical arena treating patients. At the same time, audiologists very often ask consumers to pay for elective services out-of-pocket. This element of their profession requires them to serve customers. Given this duality (Figure 1–9), audiologists must approach quality from both a medical and a retail perspective.

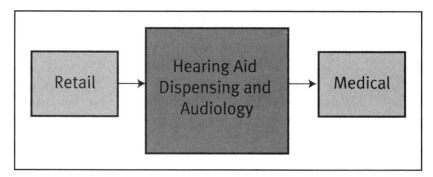

Figure 1–9. Audiology: the merging of two different worlds.

@*CONNECT*

Malcolm Baldridge and the
Baldridge National Quality Award

Malcolm Baldridge was a U.S. Representative from Nebraska and the Secretary of Commerce under President Reagan. Baldrige's award-winning managerial excellence contributed to long-term improvement in economy, efficiency, and effectiveness in government. Within the Commerce Department, Baldrige reduced the budget by more than 30% and administrative personnel by 25%. The Malcolm Baldridge National Quality Award was established in his honor in 1988. Since that time more than 300 businesses and other enterprises have been given the award.

The award promotes awareness of performance excellence as an increasingly important element in competitiveness. It also promotes the sharing of successful performance strategies and the benefits derived from using these strategies. To receive a Baldridge Award, an organization must have a role-model organizational management system that ensures continuous improvement in delivering products and/or services, demonstrates efficient and effective operations, and provides a way of engaging and responding to customers and other stakeholders.

The Baldridge National Quality Award serves two main purposes: (1) to identify organizations that will serve as role models for other organizations, and (2) to help organizations assess their improvement efforts, diagnose their overall performance management system, and identify their strengths and opportunities for improvement. In addition, giving the award helps strengthen U.S. competitiveness by:

- Improving organizational performance practices, capabilities, and results

- Facilitating communication and sharing of information on best practices among U.S. organizations of all types
- Serving as a tool for understanding and managing performance and for guiding planning and opportunities for learning

Exactly how quality gets defined largely depends on the orientation of the individual audiologist. For the medically oriented audiologist, quality may be defined as real-world outcomes with hearing aids as measured on a number of accepted self-reports (e.g., APHAB or COSI). For the retail-oriented audiologist, quality may be defined along the lines of a more financially oriented metric such as return for credit rate. In reality both views are short sighted and narrow.

In today's more competitive world, audiologists and hearing health care providers of all stripes must broaden their view of quality. By broadening their view of quality audiologists can begin the process of managing each facet of quality in their practice. Like other medical professions, audiologists have traditionally had a very narrow view of quality. This narrow view is restricted to a view of quality based on the final outcome or results of treatment, which is usually hearing aid use. On the other hand, the changing dynamics of the health care marketplace require that we have a much broader view of quality, as shown in Figure 1–10. Like the creators of Six Sigma and other quality-manufacturing techniques, broadening your definition of quality requires gathering VOC information. "Voice of customer" is a commonly heard phrase uttered by Six Sigma black and green belts. It simply refers to the fact that you are systematically gathering data directly from your customers in an attempt to improve something. For audiologists, VOC data are likely to include collecting feedback from patients on their satisfaction with hearing aids as well as their service experience in your

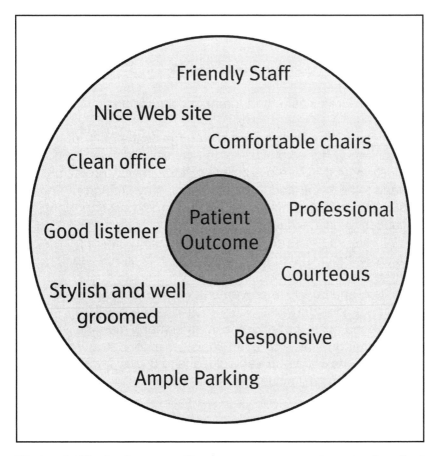

Figure 1–10. As shown, quality encompasses more than simply patient outcome.

office. When VOC data are gathered, quality can be defined in a much broader, patient-centric way. For example, patients in your clinic are just as likely to judge the results of their fitting on the friendliness of your staff, the cleanliness of your waiting room, and your bedside manner as the benefit their hearing aids provide in real-world listening conditions; therefore, audiologists need to have standards for quality for all these dimensions of the patient's experience in your clinic.

@*CONNECT*

Joseph Juran (1904–2008)

Joseph Juran was a management consultant known for applying the Pareto principle (80/20 rule) in manufacturing processes. The Pareto principle suggests that 80% of a problem is caused by 20% of the causes. Another way to think about the Pareto principle is "the vital few problems need to be separated from the trivial many problems." For quality managers this principle allows the most important causes to be identified while the outliers are ignored.

This was illustrated by his "Juran trilogy," an approach to cross-functional management, which is composed of three managerial processes: quality planning, quality control, and quality improvement. Without change, there will be a constant waste, during change there will be increased costs, but after the improvement, margins will be higher and the increased costs get recouped. Juran's applications of data-driven solutions to quality improvement were highly influential in many industries.

QUALITY FEEDBACK LOOP AND CONTINUOUS IMPROVEMENT

Quality is a data-driven process that requires discipline to implement by a team of professionals working together in a culture dedicated to self-improvement. The question for audiologists becomes how can concepts such as Six Sigma, DMAIC, root cause analysis, and the Pareto principle, which were designed for the production line, be implemented in a health care setting in which hearing aids are fitted on human beings. After all, patients are not devices. Each person brings a unique personality and set of expectations to the quality equation, for which we need to be accountable.

Once the audiologist has instilled a mindset of continuous improvement in the staff, the real work of implementing quality initiatives can begin. Using the concepts outlined in this chapter, audiologists are encouraged to follow a seven-step quality feedback loop. Since it is a feedback loop, the seven steps are continually repeated as quality outcomes are incrementally improved. No matter what aspect of quality your clinic or business is trying to improve, these seven components form the core of any quality initiative. Let us look at each component of the quality feedback loop, which is summarized in Figure 1–11:

■ Identify Things to Measure. Ask yourself the question, what needs to be improved in my clinic? There are literally dozens of processes and outcomes that can be improved in any practice, but it is best to come up with a list of three to five items. Typically, the two primary areas that can be improved revolve around the financial and clinical aspects of your practice. To keep quality initiatives feasible, it is important to narrow your list to one or two specific things in your own clinic that can improved. Once you have narrowed your list, the next step is to start seriously thinking about how you plan to measure them.

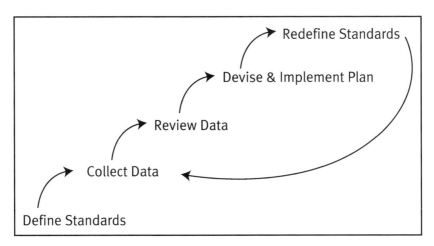

Figure 1–11. An example of a quality feedback loop is shown.

If this seems a little overwhelming, do not worry, because throughout this book we use the six steps of the patient journey as examples of what and how to measure.

■ Define Standards. The next objective is to define the standard with which you are comparing your clinic or business. Another name for a standard is "benchmark," which is a more descriptive term used to describe that with which you are comparing the data collected in your clinic. There is no shortage of published benchmarks or standards that can be applied to all realms of your practice. For example, hearing aid manufacturers may define the standard as a 10% return for credit on all products at 45 days postproduction. Audiologists could adopt that same standard when attempting to improve the return and exchange rate in their own practice. There are literally dozens of standards you could adopt for a range of procedures and outcomes. We review many of them in later chapters.

■ Collect Data. The collection of data requires that you have a tool, such as an Excel spreadsheet, checklist, and so forth. Current office management systems, such as Sycle.net, AudServ, and others, allow you to collect data on individual patients and products. Data collection systems that allow you to easily monitor data on a routine basis and mechanisms to collect and analyze the data are critical to this step. The ability to generate east-to-read reports quickly is an essential need for an office management system. Data collection systems must also allow the practitioner to easily compare data from your clinic to be compared to a benchmark. If the data in your clinic falls below the benchmark, it is a red flag that some action has to be taken by the practitioner.

■ Systematic Review of Data. The quality team reviews data on a weekly or monthly basis and compares the data collected with a standard/benchmark. The primary role of the quality team is to identify the "critical few" issues that can be improved. Once again, computerized office management system must be designed to allow practitioners the ability to quickly and efficiently review current data in relation to a benchmark or standard.

- Devise and Implement an Improvement Plan. Following a review of the data, the quality team devises and puts in place a specific plan for improving the process or outcome relative to the standard. Improvement plans must have clear action items and members of the team accountable for completing each action item must also be included in the plan.
- Identify Additional Things to Measure and Redefine Standards. As you begin to measure and improve processes and outcomes, you can begin to add things to measure and redefine benchmarks as quality improves. Once you have focused the mindset of yourself and your staff on continuous improvement and implemented this five-step process, you are well on your way to improving quality in your practice. Pat yourself on the back, because you are now creating the habit of a quality feedback loop, which leads to high-quality processes and outcomes.
- Transparency. Make results (real-world benefit, satisfaction, and return rates) available to the public. National organizations and advocacy groups could archive this information and make it available to everyone upon request.

The key take-away messages from this chapter can be summarized in the following points:

- The cornerstone of quality in the new experienced-based economy rests with your ability to sequence the patient journey along six distinct interaction stations using signature moments and memorabilia.
- Value is defined by the customer and delivered by the practitioner and staff.
- A culture and mindset of continuous improvement are needed to improve quality. This must be instilled by leaders within the organization who are willing to champion the cause.
- Business goals need to be aligned with quality initiatives.
- The entire organization is responsible for quality.
- Quality is a process that involves collecting data, analyzing gaps, and taking corrective and preventive action. It

is no longer acceptable for practitioners to ignore the implementation of best practice standards and other processes germane to quality.

Now that you have been introduced to all the essential components of quality and the patient experience model, let us dive into how to implement quality in an audiology practice.

REFERENCES

Agrawal, Y., Platz, E., & Niparko, J. K. (2008). Prevalence of hearing loss and differences by demographic characteristics among US adults: Data from the National Health & Nutrition Examination Survey, 1999–2004. *Archives of Internal Medicine, 168,* 1522–1530.

Amlani, A., & Taylor, B. (2012). Three known factors that impede hearing aid adoption rates: The influence of adoption rate reporting, marketing,and pricing strategies. *Hearing Review, 5,* 28–32.

Baker, G. (1995). *Why people buy.* New York, NY: Stendel.

Bennett, A., & O'Reilly, A. (2010). *Consumed: Rethinking business in the era of mindful spending.* New York, NY: Palgrave MacMillan.

Christensen, C. (2003). *The innovator's dilemma.* New York, NY: Harper Business.

Cotterill, A. (2011). In-store TV works: So say we all! Retrieved from http://www.dailydooh.com/

Dodson, B. (2011). Just DOOH it: How a digital reception area can enhance your practice. *Audiology Practices, 3*(2), 8–13.

Edelman, D. C. (2010). Branding in the digital age: You're spending all your money in all the wrong places. *Harvard Business Review, 11,* 63–70.

Grant-Halvorson, H. (2012). *Nine things successful people do differently.* Boston, MA: Harvard Business School Press.

Gupta, P. (2007). *Six sigma business scorecard.* New York, NY: McGraw-Hill.

Hawes, N., & Niswander, P. (1985). Comparison of the revised hearing performance inventory. *Ear and Hearing, 6,* 93–97.

Killion, M., Niquette, P. A., Gudmundsen, G. I., Revit, L. J., & Banerjee, S. (2004). Development of the quick speech-in-noise test for measuring signal-to-noise ratio hearing loss in normal-hearing and hearing-impaired listeners. *Journal of the Acoustical Society of America, 116,* 2395–2405.

Kochkin, S. (2009). MarkeTrak VIII: 25-year trends in the hearing health market. *Hearing Review, 16*(10), 23–30.

Kochkin, S. (2011). MarkeTrak VIII: Patients report improved quality of life with hearing aid usage, *Hearing Journal, 64*(6), 25–32.

Kochkin, S., Beck, D., Christensen, L., Compton-Conley, C., Fligor, B. J., Kricos, P., . . . Turner, R. G. (2010). MarkeTrak VIII: The impact of the hearing healthcare professional on hearing aid user success. *Hearing Review, 12*(4), 12–31.

Laplante-Lévesque, A., Hickson, L., & Worrall, L. (2012). What makes adults with hearing impairment take up hearing aids or communication programs and achieve successful outcomes? *Ear and Hearing, 33*(1), 79–93.

Mahdavi, S. (2011). We hate to wait. *Audiology Practices, 3*(4), 16–18.

Makary, M. (2012). *Unaccountable: What hospitals won't tell you and how transparency can revolutionize health care.* New York, NY: Bloomsbury Press.

Mueller, H. G. (2011). How loud is too loud? Using loudness discomfort level measures for hearing aid fitting and verification, part 1 and part 2. *Audiology Online.* Retrieved from http://www.audiologyonline.com/

Nabelek, A. K., Freyaldenhoven, M. C., Tampas, J. W., & Burchfield, S. B. (2006). Acceptable noise level as a predictor of hearing aid use. *Journal of the American Academy of Audiology, 17*(9), 626–639.

Palmer, C., Solodar, H., Hurley, W., Byrne, D., & Williams, K. (2009). Relationship between self-perception of hearing ability and hearing aid purchase. *Journal of the American Academy of Audiology, 20*(6), 341–348.

Pine, J., & Gilmore, J. (2011). *The experience economy* (2nd ed.). Cambridge, MA: HBS Press.

Poost-Foroosh, L., Jennings, M., & Cheesman, M. (2012). Adopting a client-centered approach for the hearing aid uptake process. *Audiology Practices, 4*(4), 10–19.

Sandridge, S., & Newman, C. (2006). Improving the efficiency and accountability of the hearing aid selection process: Use of the COAT. *Audiology Online.* Retrieved from http://www.audiologyonline.com/

Taylor, B. (2007). Audiologic predictors of hearing aid success: An evidence-based review of the literature. *Audiology Online.* Retreived from http://www.audiologyonline.com/

Taylor, B. (2009). Survey of current business practices reveals opportunities for improvement. *Hearing Journal, 62*(9), 25–31.

Taylor, B., & Bernstein, J. (2011). The red flag matrix hearing aid counseling tool. *Audiology Online.* Retrieved from http://www.audiologyonline.com/

Thibodeau, L. (2004). Maximizing communication via hearing assistance technology: Plotting beyond the audiogram! Special Issue: Assistive Listening Devices. *Hearing Journal, 57,* 46–51.

Ventry, I., & Weinstein, B. (1982). The Hearing Handicap Inventory for the Elderly: A new tool. *Ear and Hearing, 3,* 128–134.

Wilson, R. (2011). Clinical experience with the Words-in-Noise Test on 3430 veterans: Comparison with pure-tone thresholds and word recognition performance. *Journal of the American Academy of Audiology, 22,* 405–423.

2

THE THREE ESSENTIALS OF QUALITY IN AUDIOLOGY

Feeling hungry? Want to take a ride in a luxury sedan? Maybe you have the urge to put down this book and do some power shopping. Perhaps you are an executive with a Cadillac health plan that allows you to visit Rochester, Minnesota, once a year to receive a thorough medical workup from a team of physicians. (The fact that this service is referred to as a "Cadillac" plan speaks volumes for the reputation of both the health plan and the automobile after which it is named.) Before we take a deep dive into quality, let us take a few moments and look at some well-known companies outside the world of audiology. Heinz Tomato Ketchup, Lexus, Nordstrom's, and Mayo Clinic are highly regarded brands that are household names. In order to gain an appreciation for how a maniacal focus on quality affects the reputation and profitability of any organization, let us continue to discuss the underpinnings of quality by reviewing these four outstanding organizations.

Heinz Tomato Ketchup is manufactured by H. J. Heinz company. According to their Web site, it is the best known and most popular brand that the H. J. Heinz company has ever produced. Known for its difficulty coming out of the bottle—if you are over the age of 35 years, you are sure to remember "Anticipation" being sung by Carly Simon in their television commercials—more than 650 million bottles of Heinz Tomato Ketchup are sold around the world each year. Interestingly, H. J. Heinz only produces two varieties of their world-famous ketchup. One kind is "organic" and the other is simply Heinz Tomato Ketchup. Heinz Tomato Ketchup has a well-known bottle and label design. Even though it often costs 20 to 40% more than other brands of ketchup, it is by far the most popular household and restaurant brand of ketchup in the United States.

Lexus is the luxury vehicle division of Japanese automaker Toyota Motor Corporation. First introduced in 1989 in the United States, Lexus is now sold globally and has become Japan's largest-selling make of premium cars. In the early 1980s Toyota secretly began the process of creating Lexus and sold their first car with the Lexus name in 1989. Throughout the 1990s and 2000s Lexus grew to be the number one selling luxury car brand in North America. Lexus has managed to maintain their sales numbers over the past decade while launching several new models under the Lexus brand.

Nordstrom, Inc., is an upscale department store chain in the United States, founded by John W. Nordstrom and Carl F. Wallin. Initially a shoe retailer, the company today also sells clothing, accessories, handbags, jewelry, cosmetics, fragrances, and in some locations, home furnishings. There are now 225 stores operating in 29 states across the United States. Nordstrom is well known for its highly personalized customer service. The now infamous story of the local farmer mistakenly trying to return a set of tires and still getting store credit illustrates the level of customer service delivered by Nordstrom.

Nordstrom is also well known for empowering their front-line staff with a significant amount of decision-making power. In fact, until recently all new hires were given a one-page employee "handbook" with the following message emboldened on the center of the page: "Nordstrom Rule #1: Use best judgment in all situations. There will be no additional rules." This level of trust in a frontline employee's ability to do what is right for each customer has engendered a truly loyal following among Nordstrom shoppers.

Mayo Clinic is a not-for-profit medical practice and medical research group based in Rochester, Minnesota. Patients are referred to Mayo Clinic from across the United States and the world, and it is known for innovative treatments. It is also known for its team approach in which physicians are paid as employees rather than independent operators. Mayo Clinic is also known for being at the top of most accredited quality standard listings. It has been near the top of the U.S. News & World Report List of Best Hospitals for more than 20 years. Mayo Clinic is distinguished by integrated care, and a strong research presence is evidenced by the fact that over 40% of its resources are devoted to research. Mayo Clinic is also known for three core values: patient care, education, and research. The three shields on the Mayo Clinic logo signify these core values.

You do not have to enjoy ketchup on your hot dogs, own a luxury sport utility vehicle, buy a pair of $200 shoes, or make an appointment for an exam at Mayo Clinic to appreciate the lessons from these four brands. All four of these brands were started by a small group of passionate entrepreneurs who had an obsession with quality. Over time their obsession with quality of service and quality of product resulted in significant growth and profitability. Each of these organizations brings a key element of quality to our attention. The key attribute each firm is known for is summarized in Table 2–1. These key attributes are essential ingredients to the quality equation.

Table 2–1. The key attribute contributing to reputation of quality for the four brands mentioned in Chapter 2. All four attributes are essential underpinnings of quality.

Heinz Tomato Ketchup: Consistency
Lexus: Innovation
Nordstrom: Personalized Customer Service
Mayo Clinic: Unchanging Core Values

In addition to these attributes, all four brands use a continuous improvement mindset, voice-of-the-customer information, data-driven decision-making processes, and other principles discussed in Chapter 1 to continue to prosper and grow. As you will learn in this chapter, the underpinnings of quality require attention to detail and a continuous improvement mindset. These basic characteristics are what coalesce to form the foundation of quality in audiology. The purpose of Chapter 2 is to introduce you to the three universal and essential components to improving quality in a clinical audiology practice. In other words, by applying data-driven, patient-centered processes around the three essentials of quality, you will be that much closer to the goal of being known for best-in-class quality in your marketplace.

BEING A STEWARD FOR QUALITY

Movements often begin with a small group of like-minded, passionate people all pulling in the same direction over a common cause. Given the perceived need of the hearing care industry to raise the bar on quality, now is the time for a movement within the audiology and hearing instrument communities to begin. Interested professionals need to look no further than the Marke-Trak data of Sergei Kochkin for inspiration. Kochkin (2010) has intimated that approximately one-third of all hearing aid fittings result in failure. This percentage might seem quite high, but when you consider that returns for credit and in-the-drawer rates are both in double digits, one can begin to realize that quality control at the point of sale might be an issue plaguing the entire industry. In fact, Kochkin (2010) estimates that the industry has lost $69 billion in sales opportunities as a result of quality-related problems over the past two decades.

The call to action to improve quality is not confined to the MarkeTrak studies. Taylor and Rogin (2011) reported on a Hearing Industries Association (HIA) survey and found that there are opportunities to improve the way professionals deliver quality of care. Finally, in 2009, *Consumer Reports* followed a small group of patients for 6 months over their journey to purchase hearing instruments. They reported that approximately 40% of all hearing aids were "misfit." Even though virtually every industry organization, including the American Academy of Audiology, Academy of Doctors of Audiology, and the International Hearing Society, have published best practice guidelines, which are an integral part of any quality control process, they are not routinely used in clinical practice. An aim of this book is to bridge the gap between a published best practice guideline and the practicality of bringing those guidelines to life as part of a comprehensive, data-driven quality movement; the latter requires that a few bold individuals stand up and become vocal stewards for quality.

DATA-DRIVEN KEY PERFORMANCE INDICATORS

Believe it or not, major league baseball is a great example of how data are used to improve performance. Due to the high stakes nature of professional sports, baseball has been using data for measuring performance for well over 100 years. Historically, key performance indicators, such as batting average and earned run average, have been used as a metric for overall performance on the baseball diamond. Not unlike today, if the shortstop's batting average is below, say, .250, there is a good chance he will be spending more time with the batting instructor between games, than the first baseman who is hitting over .350. Batting average is an example of a commonly used key performance indicator (KPI). We actually spend a lot more time discussing KPIs in later chapters. For now, however, the main point is that data can be used to make decisions about performance. When a major league manager is making decisions about changing pitchers late in a close game, he reviews several KPIs related to how his pitching staff performs against all the batters on the other team. With the evolution of computers the amount of data that is used to make these decisions has grown by leaps and bounds. Today, the manager not only looks at the opponent's individual batting averages against his pitching staff, he also evaluates several other metrics related to the time of the game, such as weather conditions and time of day. The question for audiologists is what data will you collect that will help you make better decisions for your patients and your business?

Another lesson from Chapter 1 is that quality control is a process of continuous improvement requiring voice-of-customer information in order for the practitioner to make decisions that improve quality of outcomes. These data-driven, patient-centered decisions allow practitioners the ability to incrementally improve both the quality of care patients receive and the quality of how their businesses operate.

#DISCOVER

Common Business Key Performance Indicators for Audiologists

Return Rate—the total revenue of hearing aids returned for credit divided by the total revenue, expressed as a percentage, calculated monthly. Benchmark: 5 to 10%.

Close Rate—the total number of patients purchasing hearing aids divided by the number of opportunities, expressed as a percentage and calculated monthly. An opportunity is usually defined as a patient with a hearing loss greater than 40 dB HL (pure-tone average at 1, 2, and 4 KHz). Benchmark: 60% of opportunities should agree to purchase.

Binaural Rate—the total number of units sold divided by the total number of eligible "ears" (a patient with one "dead" ear would count as one ear, not two ears). This rate is expressed as a percentage and is calculated monthly. Benchmark: 85%.

Product Mix—a breakdown in revenue as a function of product mix. Benchmark: 20% premium, 60% business class, 20% entry level products. This KPI is highly dependent on the market which your practice is trying to attract.

The benchmarks given are relatively common, accepted standards for each KPI. It is up to the individual practice to develop their own KPIs based on data.

Over the past several years other sectors of the health care service and medical device industries have become more patient-centric and data driven. This has generally resulted in better outcomes for patients and additional profits for businesses. Recently, it seems several health care service providers have adopted many of the quality principles, such as Six Sigma, into their delivery of services. For example, physicians are now beginning to be reimbursed based on the results of their treatments, rather than the number of procedures performed and billed to insurance. There is no reason, given the economic landscape as it relates to health care, to think this trend is an aberration. It is likely that audiologists will also be adapting a results-oriented reimbursement system over the next several years. Since reimbursement systems are changing to this results-oriented model and many audiologists already practice on a direct-to-consumer "cash" basis, in which services are not billed to a third-party insurer, it is important to raise the bar on quality in order to stay competitive.

To implement a quality system into your clinical practice, there are three major components that need to be accounted for.

#DISCOVER

Baseball and Quality

If you are a cerebral baseball fan, you have probably heard the term "sabermetrics." The term is derived from an acronym for Society for American Baseball Research. The pioneer of sabermetrics is Bill James, who is famous for publishing many versions of his "Baseball Abstract." Using elaborate statistical analysis, James and other Sabermetricians use data to make judgments about performance. It serves as a good example of how data can be applied to the decision-making process. If you are looking for a way to understand the creative process of applied statistical analysis in order to apply it to the process of performance management, it might be worth checking out the work of Bill James for some inspiration.

Using the data-driven, patient-centric principles learned in Chapter 1, combined with the lessons of four well-known "quality" brands, practitioners must account for the three essential components of quality: effectiveness, efficiency, and an emphasis-on-results. Your ability to orchestrate and execute a plan around each of these three components, shown in Figure 2–1, is likely to result in your becoming the provider of choice in your marketplace. Of course, the by-products of being known as the provider of choice has many benefits to your practice, including having the luxury to command a higher selling price and more word-of-mouth referrals, which generate more revenue for your practice without your having to spend additional money on marketing. Since enjoying provider-of-choice status has benefits, let us go into detail about each of these essential components of quality.

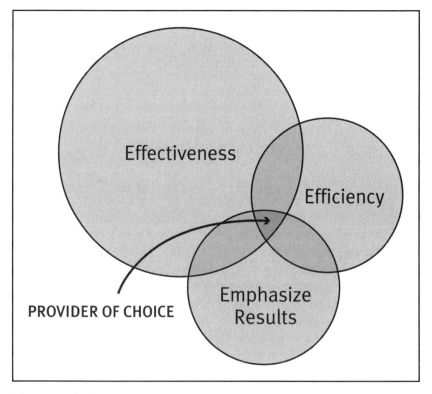

Figure 2–1. The three essentials of quality.

Effectiveness

The impact our decisions and actions have on the final result defines the term effectiveness. Being effective means that you are doing "the rights things" to contribute to a favorable patient outcome. Conducting the right tests, asking the right questions, and ordering the right hearing aids are all part of being an effective professional. Experts agree that "doing the right thing" is intertwined with the use of evidence-based practice thinking.

Your ability to incorporate relevant research findings into the clinical decision-making process is commonly known as evidence-based practice. Using evidence-based practice guidelines as part of the clinical decision-making process has a relatively short history in the annals of health care, as the topic has been taught in medical schools and subsequently applied in clinical practice for less than 30 years. In essence, the systematic approach of using relevant research as part of the clinical decision-making process ensures that our treatments will be effective. Effectiveness in an evidence-based paradigm means that our treatments and intervention provide the patient some amount of benefit and satisfaction in the real world. Much has been written about how evidence-based practice fits into the audiologist's armamentarium. One of the best review articles on the subject as it relates to audiology was published by Cox (2005). Interested readers are encouraged to seek other sources and perhaps enroll in a course on the subject of evidence-based practice. For our purposes we review the essential components of evidence-based practice from the perspective of continuous quality improvement in an audiology practice.

Evidence-based practice is a methodical six-step process that is designed to culminate in a better real-world outcome for the patient. Here are the six steps:

Step 1: Formulate a specific question that pertains to the patient and treatment option.

Step 2: Conduct a key word search using PubMed and other search engines.

Step 3: Narrow your search by reading all the abstracts and eliminating those that do not directly pertain to your question.

Step 4: Read all the articles that pertain to your question, paying particular attention to the design and power of the study.

Step 5: Evaluate or grade the quality of the evidence based on your reading of the research articles.

Step 6: Formulate a treatment option, modify a procedure, or change a behavior based on your systematic evaluation of the evidence that pertains to the question.

@CONNECT

Dr. Robyn Cox, Quality Maven

Robyn Cox's article in a 2005 issue of the *Journal of the American Academy of Audiology* is still perhaps the best short read on evidence-based principles as they relate to audiology. In addition to Cox's fine work in this area, Trisha's Greenhalgh's book, *How to Read a Paper* (Greenhalgh, 2001), is an excellent source if you wish to learn more about evidence-based practice principles.

If you are unfamiliar with how the evidence-based decision process works, you might be surprised by the amount of reading you have to do. Although evidence-based practice requires some reading, it is important to remember that *what* you read is gathered in a systematic manner. When a question is precisely formulated and the abstracts are carefully eliminated, you are usually left with a half dozen or less papers to read. Also, there are a considerable number of systematic review articles (sometimes called meta-analysis) that reduce the sheer volume of reading.

Upon initial glance, it might seem like evidence-based "thinking" and decision making requires an exceptional amount of reading. Although putting evidence-based decision making into practice does require you to stay current in your journal reading, it is wrong to assume you will be spending hours each week culling dozens of journals and search engines.

Perhaps a more critical area of evidence-based decision making is knowing how to formulate the right question that can be answered by conducting a literature search, and then knowing how to interpret the relevance of an article to a particular patient or clinical environment. Palmer, Mormer, Ortmann, Byrne, Ye, and Keogh (2008) at the University of Pittsburgh have coined the acronym REAL, which stands for Research Evaluation for Audiology Literature, as a way to think about the key attributes of evaluation of a study or research report. Let us look at the five components of how you can "stay REAL" when you are using research in the clinical decision-making process.

These five REAL components should be included in the reporting of any study published in a peer review journal, but, oftentimes, they are not. Therefore, it is up to the consumer of the research—the audiologist—to critically evaluate the quality of the research presented in the article you are reading. You can use the following five REAL points in your evaluation and grading of the quality of the research article you are reading. Here are those five REAL points:

1. Levels of Evidence

There are six distinctly different study designs, shown in Table 2–2, that the reader needs to consider. The quality of the study design can be placed into one of these six categories. The lower the number, the higher the quality of the study design. Randomized control studies, which take a group of study participants with similar characteristics and then randomly assign them to one of two groups—one group receiving "the treatment" being studied and the other group not receiving it, serve as the highest level of evidence. Randomized control trials can be contrasted with observational studies. Observational studies do not randomly assign study participants into groups, therefore there are many variables that cannot be carefully controlled in an observational study. Because of this lack of control observational studies can sometimes provide misleading results. Observational studies can still provide valuable information, but are

Table 2–2. Levels of Evidence

Level 1: Systematic reviews and meta-analyses of randomized controlled trials
Level 2: Randomized controlled trials
Level 3: Nonrandomized intervention or observational studies
Level 4: Descriptive studies (cohort studies, cross-sectional surveys)
Level 5: Case studies
Level 6: Expert opinions

a lesser level of evidence relative to randomized control trials. Obviously, you are seeking studies that have a high level of evidence, such as a level 1 or level 2 study as indicated in Table 2–2 when making an important clinical decision; however, it is relatively rare to find audiology and hearing aid research above level 3.

2. Rationale for Sample Size of the Study

The basic idea behind knowing something about the rationale for the sample size of the study allows us to set the parameters for the margin for error. Even the most well-designed study will have some margin of error. The question really is what is the allowable amount of error. The design of the study largely determines these parameters before the study is even conducted.

The sample size refers to the number of participants in the study. It is important that the sample used in the study reflect the population that you are evaluating. For example, if you are interested in the effects of noise-reduction technology in adults over the age of 70 years, you are not going to consider the findings for noise-reduction studies conducted on a young adult population.

The actual number of participants in a study is not as important as the "power" of the study. A study's power is a number between 0 and 1 are refers to the percentage of samples that are likely to be different from the sample (or lie in the region of rejection). Typically, studies that have a "power" rating of 0.8 or higher have been well designed. A study "power" of 0.8 means that if the two population samples are really different, you will find this difference 80% of the time. As a consumer of research, probably the most important question to consider relative to sample size would be to know whether or not the researchers made a "sample-size calculation" prior to conducting the research. If the "power of the study" is 0.8 or better, that is one piece of information that makes it a strong study.

Alpha level is another factor that contributes to the power of a study. The alpha score determines the significant difference between groups. Like sample size, alpha is predetermined before the study is conducted. The alpha level indicates how sure the researcher wants to be that the results do not happen by chance. An alpha of 0.03 means there is a 3% chance you will say there is a difference between treatments when there actually is no difference. Most audiology studies use an alpha between 0.01 and 0.05, which means researchers are willing to find a difference between treatments when one actually does not exist between 1% and 5% of the time.

3. Variability in the Data

The variability of the study is represented by standard deviation. Variability in the data is usually depicted on a graph of the data using standard error bars. Without the standard deviation displayed on the graph, it is impossible to know how much variability there is in the data. In fact, without the standard error bars it is impossible to know, which makes the data presented in any graph relatively meaningless.

4. Statistical and Clinical Significance

If a study is statistically significant, this means the results did not happen by chance. The parameters that determine statistical significance are set prior to the study (i.e., alpha and sample size). Evaluating the statistical significance of a study is often the first step in the interpretation of the results. If the study does not have statistical significance, you can be confident that the treatment or technology being evaluated in the study does not make a difference. Of course, this conclusion would influence a clinical decision or recommendation. For various reasons, most studies do show some degree of statistical significance; however, there might be times when it is good to know when recommendations or treatments are not different from each other. For example, if a new hearing aid technology is compared with the hearing of normal-hearing individuals, you probably do not want to see a difference between communications with hearing aids when compared with the normal-hearing listeners.

Even though a study finding might be statistically significant, it may not have practical significance in your clinic. For example, if patients who used a new type of noise-reduction technology had a 1-dB improvement on a speech-in-noise test result as compared with the group not using this feature that was deemed statistically significant, it would be virtually impossible to measure that improvement with patients in your clinic; thus, the results would not have practical significance.

5. Grade of the Study

Once all of the above factors are taken into consideration, evidence-based practice guidelines require you to assign a grade to the evidence presented in the study. These grades correspond to the level of evidence (see Table 2–2) you have assigned the study. Table 2–3 depicts the grades you may assign to studies.

Your ability to be a good consumer of research allows you to put evidence-based principles into practice. Implementation of evidence-based thinking and decision making is intended to help clinicians deliver more effective treatments. Putting evi-

Table 2–3. Grades of Evidence

A:	Consistent level 1 or 2 studies
B:	Consistent level 3 or 4 studies or extrapolations from level 1 or 2 studies
C:	Level 5 studies or extrapolations from level 3 or 4 studies
D:	Level 6 evidence or inconclusive studies from any level

dence-based principles into practice is likely to require that you enroll in a course or, at the very least, attend a seminar on the topic, as this summary is intended only to scratch the surface.

Efficiency

If being effective is about doing the right things, then being efficient is about doing the right things in the right manner. It is possible to be effective and not very efficient. Let us say that you have to cut down a large dead tree in your front yard. Since you grew up in a family of lumberjacks, you know all the steps to cutting down the tree so that it does not fall on your house; however, since you have not used your chainsaw in several years, it is not very sharp; thus, it takes you a long time to cut down the tree. This is an example of being effective, but not very efficient.

On the other hand, your neighbor who has no experience in lumberjacking, but who owns a brand new chainsaw, can drop the tree in less than a minute. The problem, however, is that he does not follow the proper techniques and ends up dropping the tree directly on his new sun porch, causing thousands of dollars of damage. This is an example of efficiency without effectiveness. After all, the tree fell in a short time, but a byproduct of this efficiency is severe damage to the house.

Efficiency is really about your ability to provide results to your patient in the optimal amount of time it takes to deliver them. Efficiency is not really about speed, it is about the time it takes to provide the best results. If we go back to the tree example, after your neighbor takes a few minutes to make the proper cuts and uses a wedge to down the tree in the proper location, he added an extra 15 minutes to the cutting time, but he was actually much more efficient because the results were optimized. With proper planning, the correct result with efficiency and effectiveness was obtained. In clinical practice efficiency is related to using the proper tools for the right amount of time to obtain the best results.

Everywhere you go these days you encounter efficiency. Automobile makers are on a constant quest to make cars more fuel efficient and builders strive to make homes and offices more energy efficient. Health care is trying to become more efficient in how they take care of patients. Fortune 500 companies hire so-called efficiency experts to reduce waste. You even hear talk of NFL teams trying to run more efficient offenses. Efficiency is about trying to work smarter, rather than harder. In our quest, however, to optimize profitability or satisfaction, while reducing the amount of wasted time or expense, it is entirely possible to create unintended consequences.

Efficiency is not limited to energy consumption and Aaron Rodgers moving the Green Bay Packers quickly down the field to score another touchdown. As farmers have employed new technologies over the past hundred or so years, food has become much more plentiful and cheaper. Like the tree falling on the house, improved efficiency has a dark side. In the case of more efficient farming, it is unprecedented amounts of obesity and diabetes due in part to the abundance of low-cost, supersized meals.

For audiologists, efficiency is really about "time over target." In other words, how much time does the practitioner need to spend with each patient to optimize outcome? From an operational perspective, time over target would entail the amount of time spent on marketing, business planning, and managing to maximize profitability. Given the complexity of patient care and management of your practice, optimizing efficiency is bound to lead to better patient care and improved profitability, but also some unintended consequences.

There are hundreds of ideas out there that can lead to better efficiency; some we cover later in this chapter. Here is one quick example from a 2009 study published in the *Journal of the American Academy of Audiology*. Catherine Palmer and colleagues asked 805 patients the following question during the prefitting intake interview:

On a scale from one to ten, one being the worst and ten being the best, how would you rate your hearing ability?

This question is a helpful way to evaluate your patient's self-perception of a hearing problem. Most audiologists talk about motivation and self-perception of a possible hearing problem with their patients, but most of us probably do not directly ask our patients to quantify it in such a way. The results of this study suggest that the answer to this one simple question have the potential to improve one facet of clinical efficiency, which is the counseling and recommendation phase of the prefitting appointment. The authors assigned participants' responses into three buckets. If the patient answered 8 to 10 (minimal hearing problems), there was less than a 20% change of each patient agreeing to acquire amplification. If the patient answered between 1 and 5 (a strong likelihood that a hearing problem is perceived), there was a better than 80% chance that each patient would acquire hearing aids. Finally, for approximately one-third of patients who responded to the question with a 6 or 7, there was a 50/50 chance that they would acquire amplification—even though this group had essentially the same pure-tone average as the patients who answered the question with a 4 or 5 rating.

As you may have guessed, quantifying the answer to that question along a 1 to 10 continuum can lead to greater efficiency in the clinic. According to this study, patients responding with an 8 to 10 answer are extremely unlikely to purchase hearing aids, so the appointment becomes more educational in nature. Patients responding with an answer between 1 and 5 can be quickly and *efficiently* brought into the hearing aid selection process. There is no need to convince these patients that they need your help; simply go to work finding the best solution to their hearing loss and lifestyle. The golden opportunity rests with the patients who responded to the question with an answer of 6 or 7. The data of Palmer, Solodar, Hurley, Byrne, and Williams (2009) suggest doing something different with this group; perhaps conducting some type of comprehensive hearing aid demonstration or in-home trial of a customized trial device would lead to increased utilization of hearing aids. Taken together, most of the patients in this bucket have a substantial hearing loss and need hearing aids. They just need a little push from you.

Of course, both patients and clinics are complex systems. The law of unintended consequences suggests that improving clinical or business efficiency to any complex system is likely to lead to some unpredictable outcomes. As you read this chapter, think about how each tool or idea could improve time over target in your practice. Automated audiometry has the potential to save a lot of time on the mundane aspects of conducting a hearing assessment. Hearing kiosks and disease-state marketing have the potential to make our marketing efforts more efficient. Changing the way you conduct a case history or the use of apps for auditory training have the potential to help you optimize time over target. All are interesting tools and concepts. Do they have an unintended downside?

The unbridled quest for better efficiency is sure to have some unintended consequences. Frederick Winslow Taylor (1856–1915) is considered the world's first efficiency expert. With the use of a stopwatch he was able to improve the overall efficiency of automobile production. This led to lower production costs and, eventually, higher pay for workers. It was his seminal ideas that fueled McDonalds obsession with counting how many burgers are flipped each hour and the phone company's penchant for monitoring the number of calls each operator is expected to handle each day. These are practices that lead to better efficiency, yet have the tendency to suck the soul out of the employees. Ultimately, the challenge for audiologists is to become more efficient while not losing the soul of our practices. That is not an entirely easy combination of tasks to juggle, but perhaps this chapter can provide some guidance.

Since a large part of efficiency is related to time spent with patients, another term we use to describe efficiency is workflow. What is the optimal amount of time to spend with patients during each stage of your clinical workflow? MarkeTrak studies can give us some insights into the optimal times for various appointment types to maximize satisfaction, and we cover that soon. First, let us take a deeper dive into efficiency. Most audiology clinics do not spend much time analyzing their workflow process to see if there is a better way to do things. The reason is that these processes and workflows are done so often that they are routine, that is, you do not even have to think about them; however, analyzing your clinic's workflow is incredibly important, especially if you are managing a larger operation within a medical practice.

There are several ways to analyze your clinic's workflow. Writing out the steps of a process or workflow is one of the easiest ways to see how your clinic is really operating. Creating a flow chart, like the one shown in Figure 2–2, is usually your best option. Flow charts help you map every step of a process to see where improvements might be made.

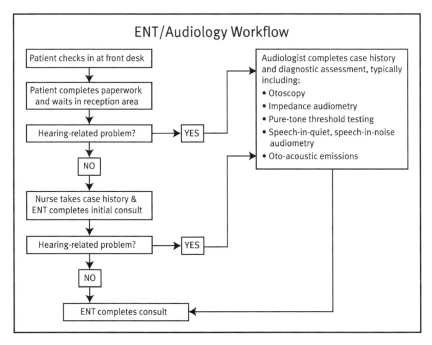

Figure 2–2. The ENT/audiology workflow is shown.

Every step gets its own box in the flow chart, and if several options are possible for a step, each option must be explored. You can get very detailed in your mapping of patient flow in your clinic. For instance, if you want to analyze patient flow in a busy ENT/audiology practice, a few of the initial flow chart steps might be as follows:

Step 1: The patient checks in.

Step 2: The patient's files are pulled and billing info is verified by front office personnel.

Step 3: Current health care eligibility is verified.

Step 4: If co-pay is required, it is collected; if not, the patient returns to the waiting room.

Step 5: The front desk lets the nurse know that the patient has arrived.

Step 6: The nurse takes the patient's records and escorts the patient to his or her room.

You get the picture. Every step of a patient's visit should be mapped out so you can see exactly what happens. As you review the steps, ask yourself why each one is done this way.

Let us turn our attention to the mapping of the workflow of a patient who is about to schedule an appointment for a "hearing problem" with an ENT/audiology practice. We skip the workflow of patient check-in at the front desk and look exclusively at the workflow from the audiologist's perspective:

Step 1: The patient calls the front office requesting an appointment.

Step 2: The front office person asks the patient a series of routine questions and books the appointment.

Step 3: Since this patient reported a possible hearing problem, two appointments are made. A 30-min appointment with the audiologist is made, followed by a 15-min appointment with the otolaryngologist.

Step 4: The audiologist brings the patient to the exam room from the reception area.

Step 5: Following greeting, the audiologist completes the case history.

Step 6: An otoscopic exam is performed.

Step 7: A brief explanation of the tests is given.

Step 8: Immittance audiometry (tymps and reflexes) is completed.

Step 9: Ear phones are inserted and the patient is instructed on the pure-tone testing procedure.

Step 10: The speech-reception threshold is obtained in both ears.

Step 11: Air conduction testing, followed by bone conduction testing, if necessary, is performed.

Step 12: Word recognition testing in quiet and noise is performed.

Step 13: The ear phones are removed and the ear tip is discarded.

Step 14: The results are discussed with patients.

Step 15: The patient is placed in a secondary waiting room to see the physician.

There you have it: a 15-step process for a 30-min appointment with the audiologist. Of course, your process might be a little different than the one shown here. The main point is that you carefully think through each step. This type of process mapping and workflow analysis can be especially important in a large practice in which several patients each day are seen by two or more professionals within the practice (e.g., an ENT/audiology practice). In smaller audiology practices, workflow analysis is still helpful. For example, as a hearing aid dispensing practice acquires more patients, it becomes inefficient to spend too much time with existing patients on follow-up and troubleshooting, while not having enough time available to see new patients. If you are finding that new patients have to wait more than a week to schedule a visit, you might want to conduct a workflow analysis to see where you are spending too much time on the wrong things.

In order to run a more efficient operation, a hearing aid practice needs to allot a specific amount of time for the common appointments that are made. Below is a list of the common appointment types made in the typical audiology practice. Along with the appointment type, notice that there is a benchmark for how long each respective appointment type should be. Using a preset amount of time for each of these appointment types is known as block scheduling. Block scheduling is common these days and most computerized office management systems allow you to do it very easily. The times you see below are based on the approximate amount of time it takes to conduct a comprehensive evaluation for each of the respective appointment types. These benchmarks are also thought to help optimize patient satisfaction, as we know from Kochkin's MarkeTrak work that there is a relationship between time spent with a patient and the patient's overall satisfaction with hearing aids.

- Hearing assessment: 30 min
- Hearing aid evaluation (combined with hearing assessment): 90 min
- Hearing aid fitting: 60 min
- Hearing aid checkup, 1 week: 30 min
- Hearing aid checkup, 1 month: 30 min
- Hearing aid check (post-trial period): 15 min for each visit

As mentioned, this technique of assigning a specific period of time for a certain appointment type is commonly known as block scheduling. It is an easy way to improve efficiency. It might seem obvious that predetermining the appointment block is a proven way to improve overall time efficiency in a practice. Of course, it is up to each practice to decide how they want to allot (or block) their times for these various types of appointments.

#DISCOVER

Process Mapping of the Patient Journey

Recall Figure 1–1 from Chapter 1. You can use the concept of process mapping and methodically record all of the steps involved in executing each of the six patient–clinician interaction stations. Ask yourself the question, "What are the 10 or so things I have to do with the patient to optimize each phase of the patient journey?" Your written response to this question forms the backbone of improving quality in your practice.

Besides appointment time, there are other issues related to efficiency. Return for credit and exchange rates are metrics that can be used to track the efficiency of your office. For example, if 20% of your patients every year are returning or exchanging their hearing aids, you have wasted a lot of precious clinical time. Chapter 5 is devoted to key business metrics, such as return for credit rates.

Let us examine the more practical aspects of efficiency. An important consideration surrounding efficiency is prioritizing how you spend your time during each of the appointment blocks you have created for your practice. Notice that the hearing assessment block is only 30 min. This means that you have a half hour to complete a comprehensive audiological evaluation of one patient. Of course, this is the *average* amount of time it will take to build rapport, take a case history, conduct several tests, and review the results. When you know a patient with special needs is being scheduled, it makes sense to simply allot more time for the appointment. More often than not, however, clinicians need to find ways to save time without compromising results. Here are some tips for saving precious clinical time without compromising accuracy and reliability during the hearing assessment time block:

- For speech audiometry, use a recorded ½ list ordered by difficulty. If the patient gets 9 or 10 of the first 10 words in the list correct, stop the test. The ordered-by-difficulty word list can be obtained from Auditec in St. Louis, MO (Hall & Mueller, 1997).
- Complete tympanometry and acoustic reflexes before the pure-tone testing. If tymps and reflexes are completely normal, skip bone conduction testing. Use insert ear phones, because in addition to the higher interaural attenuation factor relative to traditional headphones, which reduces the need to mask on some occasions, insert earphones eliminate collapsing ear canal artifact (Berlin, 2001; Hall, 2010).
- When reviewing test results, ask the patient if they want a summary of the results or a detailed explanation. Most patients will request a summary, which can be completed in about a minute.
- Look for other ways to maintain the integrity of the appointment time without compromising results. Remember that there is no better way to exude quality than "face time" with a patient. Spending a few extra minutes empathetically listening to a patient is a great way to build a

lasting bond. Time is your most valuable resource and must always be used wisely.

@*CONNECT*

The Three Essential Components of Evidence-Based Practice

As you have probably gathered from this chapter, the ability to implement evidence-based practice decision making into your clinical repertoire is imperative to improving and maintaining quality. Not to be confused with the three essentials of quality, there are also three essentials of evidence-based practice:

- Efficacy: Does the treatment provide benefit in the lab?
- Effectiveness: Does the treatment provide benefit in the real world?
- Efficiency: Is the treatment worth the money?

In an evidence-based practice paradigm, efficiency has nothing to do with time; however, the use of the term "efficiency" is about cost relative to benefit. At its core, efficiency is really a relationship between two variables. In the case of evidence-based practice it is the relationship between cost and real-world benefit. In the case of running a practice, it is the relationship between time spent with a patient and the ability to conduct an accurate and reliable assessment, or the relationship between time and revenue generated. When you think about efficiency, think about ratios.

Efficiency is really a relationship between two variables. The previous section looked at the relationship between overall time available each day (e.g., 6 hours of total appointment time) and actual time needed for various appointment types (e.g., hearing aid evaluation). Another measure of efficiency can be best classified as "time over target." In other words, how much time or

@*CONNECT*

Sergei Kochkin, Ph.D., Quality Maven

Sergei Kochkin is probably the most cited researcher in the hearing aid industry. For more than 20 years he has written dozens of papers and conducted hundreds of presentations centered around patient satisfaction. Many of you might know him as the man behind the MarkeTrak studies. His research is a rare example of work in the area of clinical quality and much of it is cited throughout this book. Here is what Sergei has to say about hearing loss and hearing aids:

> Society in general views hearing loss as a benign condition. It is not hearing loss per se that is the problem. It is the problem that hearing loss causes you in your experience as a human being. Research demonstrates the considerable negative social, psychological, cognitive and health effects of untreated hearing loss . . . with far-reaching implications that go well beyond hearing alone. In fact, those who have difficulty hearing can experience such distorted and incomplete communication that it seriously impacts their professional and personal lives, at times leading to isolation and withdrawal. Studies have linked untreated hearing loss to: irritability, negativism and anger; fatigue, tension, stress and depression; avoidance or withdrawal from social situations; social rejection and loneliness; reduced alertness and increased risk to personal safety; impaired memory and ability to learn new tasks; reduced job performance and earning power; diminished psychological and overall health.
>
> Hearing aids are miniature electronic marvels which can now be programmed to precisely meet the needs of most people with hearing loss. It's a mistake to think that you can take them out of the box like they came from Best Buy, pop them in your ears, and you will hear and understand like you can see when putting on glasses. The successful hearing aid journey is dependent on finding a hearing health professional who uses best practices in fitting your hearing aids.

how many appointments are needed, on average, to optimized satisfaction for each patients. According to Kochkin (2011) 76% of patients with above-average success were fit in one or two visits compared with 40% of patients who experienced below-average success with amplification. Furthermore, 47% of patients with below-average success required four to six visits to fit their devices compared with 7% of patients who experienced above-average success with the same number of office visits. Kochkin (2011) determined that verification and validation procedures, which generally entail the use of probe-microphone measures and self-reports of outcome, result in fewer office visits to obtain a favorable result. Specifically, the use of both verification and validation of a fitting leads to 2.41 average patient visits, while conducting neither validation nor verification leads to 3.57 average patients visits. One could conclude that the use of current verification and validation procedures results in 1.2 fewer visits for each patient receiving new hearing aids. When these "time-over-target" figures are applied to an entire year of appointment times, it becomes obvious that the use of both verification and validation procedures leads to a much more efficient office. In the next chapter, we address specific procedures or "best practices" that lead to more clinical efficiency, and thus higher-quality patient outcomes.

EMPHASIS ON RESULTS

A significant portion of quality is related to measuring results. The term "result" is used very broadly here, as a relatively small, but very important part of getting a good "result" is the benefit and satisfaction of the patient. Other aspects of the patient's experience in your clinic also have a result associated with them. For example, there is a result associated with your marketing efforts, of the wait in your reception and even a result of the patient's interaction with your staff. All of these are important aspects of quality that can be measured. This section provides some insight into how many of these "results" can be measured.

You may have noticed the word "benchmark" in the previous section and wondered what it meant. Benchmark is another word for a standard. Benchmarks are often needed to measure results. A benchmark (or standard) is used to compare the performance or result of an important variable in your business. The term presumably originates from the practice of making dimensional height measurements of an object on a workbench using a graduated scale or similar tool, and using the surface of the workbench as the origin for the measurements. You don't have to be a carpenter to appreciate that the process of benchmarking involves using best practice information and comparing it with variables in your own practice. In order to conduct benchmarking you need two things. First, you must have best practice information. The term "best practice" implies that you are benchmarking against what is considered "best in class" for a particular variable. Often, it is difficult or even impossible to know what is "best in class." When true best practice information is not available, survey data can be used as a means of comparison. Using survey data typically means you are comparing with an average of several clinics.

Second, in order to make a comparison you need to measure the variable in your office. It has been said that in order to improve something you must first find a way to measure it. The act of measuring something implies that you understand the result. For example, there are several ways to measure the result of a hearing aid fitting. From a business standpoint, the average sales price and return for credit rate are ways to gauge the result of your business. Obviously, these are important variables to measure, and we cover them in detail in Chapter 5. Keep in mind, however, that quality initiatives must be patient-centric, which requires that results be measured in different ways; therefore, let us take a closer look at how the results of a patient's experience in your clinic can be measured.

In general, there are two ways to measure anything. The most common way to measure is directly. A direct measure is one in which the outcome is compared with a specific benchmark. There are several direct measures of quality. Comparing the output, gain, and distortion of a hearing aid in your 2-cc coupler with an American National Standards Institute (ANSI) standard is a direct measure of hearing aid performance. If your coupler measure deviates more than 3 dB from the ANSI standard, then you are likely to send the hearing aid back to the manufacturer.

#*DISCOVER*

Practice Benchmarks

Over the past few years (beginning in 2010) Phonak has sponsored an annual survey of key metrics in hearing aid dispensing practices. By surveying hundreds of practices around the United States, they provide baseline information for several key performance indicators. Since such a diverse range of practices are surveyed, practices can easily compare several variables in their practice with the median. In many cases, by looking at the top 20% of those surveyed, you can even generate some comparisons in your clinic with "best practices" that may be employed by practices similar to yours. Since a significant component to quality is the use of benchmarks to measure certain key performance indicators against a standard, these survey data are extremely useful. To obtain your copy of Phonak's annual study, contact your local Phonak representative.

Another example of a direct measure would be word recognition scores. If a patient scores 92% on the NU-6 word list, that tells you that the patient has an excellent ability to understand speech in quiet relative to the NU-6 normative data. Direct measures of quality provide objective information about performance. Since direct measures provide a quantifiable score or result, they are generally straightforward to measure. Simple and straightforward scores provide us with reasonable insights into hearing aid performance, but oftentimes these objective measures fail to capture the nuances of quality; therefore, indirect measures of quality are needed.

Indirect or proxy measures are used to ensure that a specific procedure or task was completed successfully. Since quality is especially difficult to measure directly, proxies are needed. Tracking sheets, protocol checklists, and patient comment cards are examples of proxy measures. Proxy measures are needed to capture many of the more intangible, almost indefinable aspects of quality. For example, a proxy measure is needed to measure many components of the six patient–provider interaction stations shown in Figure 1–1.

Proxy measures can be a bit tricky to manage. Since they are often based more on observation from your staff and rely on subjective impressions, they may not necessarily accurately reflect reality. The effective use of proxy measures in your practice require that you first set clear guidelines and expectations. Second, you must educate your staff on how to conduct specific procedures that you are measuring with a proxy. Finally, as the manager, it is your responsibility to monitor results. In other words, inspect what you expect. Proxy measures can be highly effective ways of measuring quality when you have to communicate the standards, train your staff on the proper behaviors, and provide ongoing feedback to improve performance.

@CONNECT

Van Halen and Brown M&Ms

One of the most ingenious examples of a proxy measure comes from the world of rock-and-roll. If your formative years were the 1980s, you might remember the infamous Monsters of Rock concerts. There was no shortage of pyrotechnics during these arena rock concerts and the musicians and fans were at risk if they were not properly constructed. Van Halen came up with the idea of using M&Ms as a proxy measure of a properly constructed stage. In their contract it stated that they could refuse to perform, if there were brown M&Ms in the backstage candy bowl. The brown M&Ms, or lack thereof, served as a proxy. If the band saw brown M&Ms, this was a red flag that the stage had to be more carefully inspected prior to that evening's show. After all, if the workers did not take the time to read the clause about brown M&Ms, they may have not taken the time to carefully set up the fireworks to be set off during the first set. Who knew proxy measures could be learned from a California rock band!

MEASUREMENT TOOLS

Carpenters rely on a tape measure and fish mongers rely on a scale. The purpose of these measurement tools, of course, is to ensure they are doing their jobs correctly, abiding by specific standards and conducting business in a transparent fashion. Audiologists can use certain tools for measurement for the same purposes. In order to effectively measure quality in your clinic, audiologists must rely on a variety of measurement tools; thus, a combination of direct and proxy measures can be used. Let us bring the concept of direct and proxy (indirect) measures of quality to life by discussing the seven dimensions of quality that need to be measured. Of course, there is an abundance of things you can measure in your clinic. If you have not routinely measured anything in the daily operation of your clinic, these seven things can be quite easily measured.

In-Person Greeting at Your Clinic and Wait Time

How the patient was greeted when they arrived at your office can be measured with a tracking sheet like the one shown in Table 2–4. The proxy measure is "appropriate greeting" as it implies that once it is checked off on the tracking sheet, it was done correctly. This also assumes that you have trained your staff regarding what entails an appropriate greeting. Another indirect

Table 2–4. Tracking Sheet for Appropriate In-Person Greeting and Wait Time

Patient Name	Time Arrived	Appropriate Greeting	Wait Time	Notes

measure that can be used to ensure a patient has been properly greeted by the front office staff is the "happy patient" proxy. Here is how it works: When the audiologist calls a patient from the reception area to the exam room, observe the mannerisms of the patient. If the patient is smiling and exhibiting a pleasant demeanor, that is a proxy for a good experience with the front office staff. The goal of the front office staff is to do everything possible from the greeting to the wait time in the reception area to ensure the patient is in a good mood prior to the appointment with the audiologist. The manager could establish a benchmark of 90% happy patients prior to the appointment with the audiologist and measure it with a tally of the "happy patient" proxy.

Another tracking sheet can be used to monitor greetings over the phone. Table 2–5 shows a tracking sheet that can be used to measure how patient's phone calls are converted into appointments and eventually into sales. These are important business proxies that we address in more detail in Chapter 4.

Initial Experience in the Reception Area

The quality of the patient's experience in the reception area can be measured with a checklist like the one shown in Table 2–6. This proxy measure of quality gauges the appearance of your practice. On a weekly basis this checklist can be completed by the front office assistant or manager in order to identify any

Table 2–5. Key Performance Variables at the Front Desk That Can Be Managed with a Tracking Sheet

Phone Call Conversion Tracking Sheet
No. of calls _____
No. of scheduled appointments _____
No. of kept appointments _____
No. of companions attending appointment _____
No. of units sold _____

Table 2–6. Physical Location Checklist

Date: _____ Responsible Party: _____	
Restroom is clean and stocked	
Current, tatter-free reading material in reception area	
Clean floors, walls, windows	
Furniture is clean and properly arranged	
Literature with practice brand is prominently displayed	
Well lit (no burned-out bulbs)	
No odors	
Equipment is orderly and dust-free	
Staff is properly groomed and wearing appropriate attire	
Deficient Areas:	

problems with the physical location of the clinic. Notice that the date and person responsible for completing the checklist are at the top of the form.

People Skills of the Provider

The interpersonal communication skills of the clinician can be measured with a comment card. Using a 1 to 5 Likert scale, or a 0 to 10 scale, like the one shown in Figure 2–3, you can measure

Customer Satisfaction Survey

We value your comments. Your feedback is important to us....

	◄Strongly Agree			Neutral				Strongly Disagree ►
1. The receptionist was warm, friendly and professional.	10 9 8 7	6 5	4	3 2 1	0
2. My services began in a reasonable amount of time.	10 9 8 7	6 5	4	3 2 1	0

My audiologist or hearing care professional:

3. listened to me	10 9 8 7	6 5	4	3 2 1	0
4. was knowledgeable	10 9 8 7	6 5	4	3 2 1	0
5. adequately explained the results	10 9 8 7	6 5	4	3 2 1	0
6. solved or offered solutions for my hearing needs	10 9 8 7	6 5	4	3 2 1	0
7. I am satisfied with the overall Sonus experience.	10 9 8 7	6 5	4	3 2 1	0

	◄Extremely Likely			Neutral				Not at all likely ►
8. How willing are you to recommend a family member or friend to this office?	10 9 8 7	6 5	4	3 2 1	0

9. How did you hear about us? (please circle one)

newspaper ad   mail   family/friend
physician   repeat visit   other: _____

Name _____

Date of visit _____

How long have you used your current hearing aids? _____

Sonus®
Hearing Care Professionals

For office use only:
APPOINTMENT TYPE (please circle)
DHT   HAE   HAD   HACK
6 month check   Annual Check
Walk-In
Location: _____

1783 FORM

Figure 2–3. An example of a comment card that measures patient satisfaction. Reprinted with permission of Sonus, Inc. Plymouth, MN.

the key behaviors of yourself and your staff, as they interact with patients. This is a good example of the type of questions to ask on a comment card. Note how many of the questions listed on the comment focus on the interpersonal skills of the clinical staff. The last question on the comment card, which asks the patient about their willingness to recommend, has been shown by Fred Reichheld of the Bain Group to be correlated with patient satisfaction. Reichheld has developed something called the Net Promoter Score, which can be calculated by dividing the total number of net promoters (circled 9 or 10 on the comment card) into the total number of scores received that are 8 and below.

@CONNECT

Fred Reichheld

Fred Reichheld is an American author and business strategist best known for his research and writing on the loyalty business model and loyalty marketing. His most recent book is *The Ultimate Question 2.0: How Net Promoter Companies Thrive in a Customer-Driven World*. He developed the Net Promoter Score (NPS), a concept based on his research in measuring customer satisfaction, customer retention, and its link to revenue growth and profitability.

Comment cards are an excellent way to measure overall customer satisfaction. An important consideration is when to ask a patient to complete a comment card or survey. MarkeTrak tells us that simply asking a patient to complete a survey improves satisfaction. In a competitive market that is reason enough to conduct a survey using a comment card. Although there seems to be no best point in time in the patient's journey to administer a survey, it makes sense to pick a couple of specific points to give out a comment card. One reasonably good time to give your patients a comment card to complete would be approximately 6 months after the fitting. By the 6-month mark, after the patient has been wearing hearing aids awhile, it seems more logical that you will receive a candid response about overall impressions of both the hearing aid performance and opinions about the service quality you are providing.

Another important consideration is how you administer the comment card to your patients. There are three ways to get the card in the hands of your patient. You can leave a stack of comment cards in your office encouraging patients to fill them out and drop them in a box. You can mail the comment cards to them, and using a postage-paid card, you have the cards mailed back to you. The third alternative would be to use a virtual comment card. This means that you allow patients to post comments on your Web site. Commonly referred to as "online reputation management" you can encourage patients to post comments on your Web site. Once you approve the comment, it can be posted on your website for others to view. This type of service is usually offered as part of a Web site package that a third party can administer for you.

Technical Skills of the Provider

The technical skills of the clinician can be measured with a protocol checklist. One way to ensure that key tests and procedures are completed is through the use of a checklist. Figure 2–4 shows a list of the clinical best practices that are expected to be conducted with each patient. It is the responsibility of each

Tests defined in the standard	Differences in Standards	
	1996	2003
Full on gain (HFA FOG)	run at 50 or 60 dB SPL	run at 50 dB SPL
Maximum output (HFA OSPL90)	AGC set by mfg suggestion	AGC set to min effect
Frequency response	at 50 or 60 dB SPL	at 60 dB SPL
Equivalent input noise	gain at 60 dB SPL	gain at 50 dB SPL
Harmonic distortion	AGC set by mfg suggestion	AGC set to min effect
Battery drain	AGC set by mfg suggestion	AGC set to min effect
Telephone coil sensitivity	AGC set by mfg suggestion	AGC set to min effect
AGC input/output	AGC set by mfg suggestion	AGC set to max effect
AGC attack and release time	AGC set by mfg suggestion	AGC set to max effect

Figure 2–4. Differences in standards are shown for 1996 and 2003.

clinician to check them off on this list after each of them has been completed with the patient. Following the appointment, the completed checklist is placed into the patient's chart or scanned into their electronic record.

@CONNECT

Dr. Gawande and *The Checklist Manifesto*

Atul Gawande, a prominent surgeon and author in Boston, wrote *The Checklist Manifesto* in 2009. His book illustrates several cases in which a checklist improves quality. Checklists in the construction, airline, and medical arenas serve as excellent examples of how results can be improved when checklists are diligently followed. *The Checklist Manifesto* is a must read for anyone skeptical about the use of checklists as a quality control measure.

Product Quality

The overall quality of the hearing instruments can be measured with an objective standardized measure. Before any hearing aid leaves the manufacturing facility, it is typically placed on a 2-cc coupler and tested to insure that it closely approximates a series of standards. Currently, the industry looks at ANSI S3.22 2003 as the standard for hearing aid performance in a 2-cc coupler. This is shown in Table 2–7. The overall quality and reliability of hearing aids can be judged with the ANSI standard. As an objective measure of quality control, clinicians are encouraged to repeat this measure in their hearing aid test box using the appropriate coupling before the hearing aids are fitted to the patient.

Use Time of the Device

Another objective measure of quality is use of the devices, as there are some data suggesting a relationship between how

Table 2–7. An Example of a Protocol Checklist

Standard	Clinical Tool/Procedure
Pretest communication assessment	• Case History • COSI • COAT • HHIE
Test	• Audiogram (air and bone) • Immittance audiometry • Speech audiometry (quiet and noise)
Post-test	• Reviewed test results • Demonstrated new technology • Discussed options • Offered recommendation

COSI, Client Oriented Scale of Improvement; COAT, Characteristics of Amplification Tool; HHIE, Hearing Handicap Inventory for the Elderly.

many hours per day the patient is wearing hearing aids and overall patient satisfaction. Data logging can be used to objectively measure how many hours per day on average a patient is wearing his or her hearing aids. Most hearing aid software allows clinicians access to not only how many hours per day the patient is wearing their hearing aids, but also precisely how long the patient is wearing their devices in the various programs or memories each day.

Benefit and Satisfaction

A lot has been written about benefit and satisfaction as it relates to hearing aid use. Since providing hearing aid benefit and patient satisfaction is probably our highest priority, an entire chapter of this book is devoted to how it can be measured in a busy clinical environment. For now, let us agree that the combination of satisfaction and benefit are one of seven things we can routinely measure in our clinic. Chapter 4 goes into detail on measurement of benefit and satisfaction of hearing aid fittings.

SEVEN THINGS TO REMEMBER ABOUT QUALITY

Seven is a lucky number for a lot of superstitious people. There are seven natural wonders of the world, seven seas, and seven dwarfs (of Snow White). There are even seven dimensions of quality that can be measured in an audiology clinic. Keeping with the theme of seven, let us look at some of the practical aspects of raising the bar on quality. Most of us work in practices that require us to ask patients to spend their hard-earned money for the products and services were offer. This forces us to be forthright and honest about how we approach the competitive commercial marketplace. The first two chapters are intended to provide a solid foundation for how a data-driven culture devoted to quality drives long-term success, improves patient benefit, and increases word-of-mouths referrals. As we move into the next three chapters, more details about how to improve quality in an audiology practice will be explored. In the meantime, here are seven things to remember about quality:

1. Quality is both rational and emotional. The best way to describe the difference between the rational and emotional aspects of quality is to think about the term "sticker shock" when purchasing a car. When you take a European sports coupe for a test drive you fall in love with the rev of the 540 horsepower engine, how it so effortlessly handles curves at 80 MPH, and the smell of the leather seats. Maybe you love it so much you decide to buy it. When you get the car home and the adrenalin rush wears off, you begin thinking about the poor gas mileage, high insurance rates, and what else you can do with the $50,000 you just borrowed from the bank. That is the interplay between the emotions and logical sides of buying. The same applies to how customers perceive the quality of your product or service. Accounting for them in your quality initiatives is important. You can have a higher-quality fitting with superior patient outcomes (logical) and poor satisfaction (emotional), and vice versa.

2. Behavior = Performance = Results. This three-word equation summarizes the essentials of results. If you want superior results, you need superior performance, and if you want superior performance, the foundation is superior behaviors. The equation also serves to remind us that behavior—the

moment-to-moment interaction with the patient—drives higher outcomes.

3. "What you do" (the functional) and "how you do it" (mechanical and humanistic) are equally important. How you complete a task or procedure with a patient is just as important as the task itself. Again, this serves to remind us that your behavior determines success.

4. Little things (details) make a big difference in perceptions of quality. In any high margin low volume business, such as hearing aid dispensing, small, seemingly meaningless details can make a huge difference in outcomes. This is especially important during the initial phases of the patient's journey before a solid relationship has been built. For example, how you ask a person for the sale at the end of an appointment can made a big difference in the outcome. Simply changing a few words or putting more emphasis on a certain word can make all the difference.

5. Many people are willing to pay more for quality. After carefully segmenting your market you are likely to find that there are a relatively large number of customers who are willing to pay a little more if the quality is better. This statement holds true for just about every product and service, including hearing aids.

6. Quality can be measured. You learned in this chapter that at least seven dimensions of quality can be measured using a combination of direct and proxy measures.

7. Only when quality is measured can it be improved. Robert Boyle, the scientist, and Peter Drucker, the business management guru, came upon the insight that when something is measured, it can be improved. That profound insight tells us that one of the primary steps in delivering the highest quality of care begins with your ability to select and measure the right things. If you are looking for right things to measure in your practice, a good place to start would be the seven dimensions of quality mentioned in this chapter.

BEST PRACTICES

Most of us are familiar with the term "best practices." It is a term used to describe the process in which the tasks and procedures recognized as being most effective are disseminated to a wider audience. To true quality experts (e.g., Six Sigma Green Belts) best practice processes are a little sloppy because without proper data collection and analysis, it is virtually impossible to define what "most effective" means. In any event, with the paucity of clinical research substantiating the effectiveness of various recommendations and procedures, best practice "thinking" is a useful approach to improving quality. Although anecdotal by definition, best practices give us the best chance of improving quality of outcomes when little systematic clinical evidence is available. Here is a five-step approach to best practice implementation. In Chapters 3 and 4 we apply these steps to building a common-sense best practice protocol for an audiology clinic:

1. Identify clinicians who provide the highest outcomes.
2. Study what these clinicians are doing.
3. Standardize these procedures.
4. Scale these standards across all practices.
5. Execute the best practices in your clinic.

Take a page from Heinz Ketchup, Lexus automobiles, Nordstrom department stores, and Mayo Clinic, and begin the process of becoming known as *the* quality provider for hearing care in your area. You can even think of what each of these companies excels at as a "best practice" that might be scaled and applied to your own practice. These well-known and successful companies have shown that when you become known for high quality, you can command a higher average selling price for your goods and services, as well as a larger share of business that comes from word-of-mouth referrals. Applying the three essentials of quality to a best practices approach is a great place to start.

REFERENCES

Berlin, C. (2001). Four tests are mandatory—and so is the order. *Hearing Journal, 54*(4), 26.

Cox, R. (2005). Evidence-based practice in provision of amplification. *Journal of the American Academy of Audiology, 16,* 419–438.

Greenhalgh, T. (2001). *How to read a paper: The basics of evidence based medicine* (2nd ed.). London, UK: BMJ Press.

Hall, J. W. (2010). Aural immittance measures are more useful now than ever. *Hearing Journal, 63*(4), 10–15.

Hall, J. W., & Mueller, H. G. (1997). *Audiologists' desk reference: Diagnostic audiology—principles, procedures and practices* (Vol. 1). San Diego, CA: Singular.

Kochkin, S. (2011). MarkeTrak VIII: Reducing patient visits through verification and validation. *Hearing Review, 18*(6), 17–18.

Kochkin, S., Beck, D., Christensen, L., Compton-Conley, C., Fligor, B. J., Kricos, P., . . . Turner, R. G. (2010). MarkeTrak VIII: The impact of the hearing healthcare professional on hearing aid user success. *Hearing Review, 12*(4), 12–31.

Palmer, C., Mormer, E., Ortmann, A., Byrne, D., Ye, Y., & Keogh, L. (2008). Is it REAL? Research evaluation for audiology literature. *Hearing Journal, 61*(10), 17–28.

Palmer, C., Solodar, H., Hurley, W., Byrne, D., & Williams, K. (2009). Relationship between self-perception of hearing ability and hearing aid purchase. *Journal of the American Academy of Audiology, 20*(6), 341–348.

Taylor, B., & Rogin, C. (2011). The top 10 ways to create consumer delight with hearing aids: Improving quality at the point of sale to establish a patient-driven practice. *Hearing Review, 7*, 12–16.

3

BEST PRACTICES AND OUTCOME MEASURES IN THE CLINIC

INTRODUCTION

The primary "take-away" from the first two chapters of this book is that audiologists must adapt a data-driven, continuous improvement culture, if they strive to deliver a high quality of care to patients and maintain a competitive advantage relative to direct-to-consumer devices. In order to implement these concepts clinicians and managers must begin this process by clearly defining and tracking their own key performance indicators. This chapter puts into action many of the principles discussed in the first two chapters by offering specific guidance on how to implement several of the best practices that are thought to lead to improved patient outcomes. The first section of the chapter addresses several tests and procedures (many of them supported by evidence) that can be used clinically. In addition to providing a list of best practices, this chapter goes into many of the details of *how* to actually conduct many of these best practices in your clinic. The second half of the chapter delves into specific measures of benefit and satisfaction that can be employed to monitor quality of outcomes. The main point is that the data you collect from patient outcome self-reports (questionnaires) can be used to make improvements to the best practices in your own clinic.

The implementation of a best practice protocol combined with the use of self-report outcome measures forms the basis for the term "reality-based practice," which is used to describe the methodology behind implementing evidence-based thinking into the delivery of high-quality care. Using the data collected in various self-reports of outcome to drive incremental improvements in how care is delivered to patients forms the cornerstone of quality in a reality-based-practice paradigm. Recall from Chapter 2 that evidence-based practice is a step-by-step decision-making process requiring the clinician to frame the proper question, conduct a review of the relevant literature, as well as grade the quality of the published studies and apply this to their decision-making process. Undoubtedly, this methodology contributes to improved decision making and ultimately higher quality of care for patients. Clinicians should continue to rely on evidence-based decision-making processes whenever possible by framing the right questions, conducting literature reviews, and generally being good consumers of the pertinent research. The challenge, however, is that many important clinical questions are difficult to answer solely through the use of evidence-based-practice methods. Research, especially of the peer-reviewed variety, often lags far behind technology advances in hearing aids. This makes it nearly impossible to make decisions using evidence-based principles when studies evaluating a specific feature in question have not been published yet. An additional challenge associated with applying evidence-based principles to the clinical decision-making process is the paucity of research that has been published on the population in question. If you are working in the commercial market and your clientele is typically between the ages of 70 and 85 years, it is important that you are reviewing and grading research on clinical questions that has been conducted on this cohort of individuals. Unfortunately, the majority of studies conducted in audiology have not been done on individuals who obtained their hearing aids in the commercial market; thus, extrapolating their results can be somewhat dubious.

Evidence-based-practice principles are certainly important, but in the face of limited research, another approach is needed.

Reality-based practice is the term that describes the bridging of evidence-based-practice principles with the needs of a busy clinic. Figure 3–1 represents the essential processes surrounding reality-based practice, with evidence-based-practice at its core. Reality-based practice relies on clinicians using "best practices" often published by expert panels representing a national professional organization and putting them into action using a protocol and data collection. Although expert opinion represents the lowest level of evidence in an evidence-based-practice paradigm, for the average clinician trying to act in the interests of their patients, best practices are a way to ensure your patients are receiving the highest quality of care when there is a shortage of level 1 to 3 evidence that can be used in the clinical decision-making process.

Since the implementation of best practice guidelines represents a significant opportunity for clinicians to standardize clinical processes, let us jump into the details of getting best practice initiatives off the ground. Before delving into some audiology "best practices" you can use in your own clinic, it is prudent to review the state of the industry with respect to the use of best

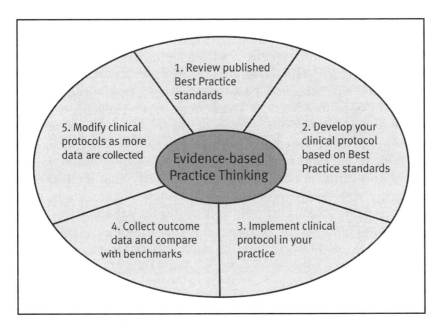

Figure 3–1. Reality-based practice is shown.

practices. After all, if market penetration were strong, patient satisfaction high, and return for credit rates low, the industry might not have any significant challenges with respect to quality. As we will discuss, however, data suggest that clinical audiology and hearing aid dispensing face several challenges with respect to quality; thus, there is considerable room for improvement.

Hartley, Rochtchina, Newall, Golding, and Mitchell (2010) surveyed 2,956 individuals between the ages of 49 and 99 years living in the Blue Mountains of Australia. Their results showed that 24.3% of hearing aid owners never wear their devices. This suggests a failure rate of nearly one in four (that is, if you consider obtaining hearing aids and never using them a "failure"). Although cost and stigma are certainly reasons for not using hearing aids, a lack of quality control is considered an obstacle to this nonuser rate. As Gopinath et al. (2011) suggest, earlier and more effective interventions could encourage older people who otherwise lack self-motivation to obtain hearing aids. It certainly seems intuitive that higher quality standards and widespread implementation of best practices would be considered "more effective" types of intervention and warrant our collective attention. Perhaps the best source for evidence supporting the need for quality improvements in the delivery of audiology and hearing aid services comes from MarkeTrak. As many people know, MarkeTrak surveys are sponsored by the Better Hearing Institute (BHI), which receives its funding from the Hearing Instrument Association (HIA). MarkeTrak consumer surveys have been conducted since the late 1980s. Since MarkeTrak surveys thousands of households every 4 years or so, it represents the best voice-of-customer information available to all interested parties; thus, MarkeTrak is the type of voice-of-customer data needed for us to raise the bar on quality.

Among the important trends that MarkeTrak periodically reports are market penetration, adaption rates, hearing loss prevalence, demographic trends, and customer satisfaction. Since the overall quality of a fitting is related to customer satisfaction, these ratings certainly would be germane to our discussion about quality in the clinic. According to MarkeTrak approximately 6 of 10 people are either "satisfied" or "very satisfied" with their hearing aids, and about 50% would repurchase their hearing aids if another set were needed. Interestingly, these scores would be considered relatively low by most quality standards. Additionally, with respect to quality standards, Kochkin (2011) reports an estimated one-third failure rate. When returns for credit, nonuse, and low use (<2 hr per day) are factored together, the failure rate indeed approximates 33%. The work of the Blue Mountains (Australia) group and Kochkin provides us with the evidence we need that quality can be improved in the dispensing of hearing aids. The question, however, remains, how do we build standardization into our clinical routines using best practice guidelines? After all, there has been no shortage of best practice standards and guidelines available to audiologists over the past several decades. The American Speech and Hearing Association (ASHA) has published several iterations of a best practice guideline for fitting adults with hearing aids (along with several pediatric guidelines), and the well-known Vanderbilt Reports published in the 1980s are another example of a clinical protocol for the purposes of fitting adults with hearing aids. Robert Margolis and colleagues at the University of Minnesota published a clinical protocol handbook in the 1990s. Several university clinics post their hearing aid selection and fitting protocol on-line (a good one comes from the University of Memphis Hearing Aid Research Laboratory). Finally, the Independent Hearing Aid Fitting Forum (IHAFF) created a protocol in 1994 that serves as yet another example of a clinical guideline.

THE HABIT LOOP

Perhaps a better question is why have not clinicians embraced the myriad of best practice guidelines that have been available to them over the past several decades? The answer to this question is probably complex, but one explanation is probably related to how people develop habits. If you think about it, a lot of the procedures and routines in which we engage with patients in the clinic are nothing more than a series of behaviors. A series of behaviors that are committed to memory and executed on a daily basis without thinking about them is one definition of a habit. Recent research on habit formation (summarized by Duhigg, 2012) suggests that habits are important because they help us conserve our efforts in order to focus on novel information. Through the formation of a habit, the prefrontal cortex of our brain is freed up to think about things that are of greater overall importance or value. For example, driving your car to work is a quite complex activity. You need to back out of your garage, navigate a busy highway, find the location of your workplace, and locate a place to park your car; however, after just a few days you do not have to consciously think about any of those tasks. Instead of consciously thinking about the drive to work, it becomes so routine that you can even start thinking about your first patient during the commute. It is as if your brain is on auto-pilot for the commute and actively thinking about your first patient of the day. According to Duhigg, activities are transferred from the prefrontal cortex to the basal ganglia when habits are formed; thus, the intellectual centers of the brain "go to sleep" and do not really think about the habit that has been committed to memory. Believe it or not, conducting everyday clinical routines, such as hearing evaluations and hearing aid fittings, are a lot like driving your car to work. The initial phases of learning these new procedures in graduate school is extremely taxing for the prefrontal cortex, but once you learn the procedures by actually doing them you do not have to think too much about them. That is an indication that your brain has moved the thinking from the prefrontal cortex to the basal ganglia. The upside to forming these habits (clinical procedures) is that it takes less mental energy to complete them. It allows you to pay more attention to any important differences you may observe for the individual you may be working with at the moment. The downside of habit formation is that once you develop a habit it is very difficult to change. Once you learn to complete a comprehensive battery of tests in a certain way, for example, it is difficult to modify or change these procedures—even when we may consciously know there is a better way to complete them!

According to Duhigg, the Habit Loop, which is shown in Figure 3–2, has three components. The cue is a trigger for the brain to go into automatic mode. The routine is the physical action that occurs after the cue has been observed. Finally, the reward is something pleasurable or stimulating to you. In the clinic the cue could be a patient eagerly waiting to see you, the routine is the hearing evaluation appointment, and the reward is

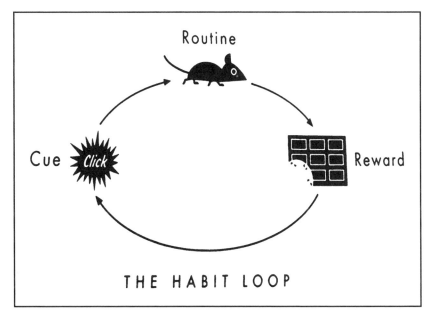

Figure 3–2. Habit Loop from Flex slides is shown.

the patient accepting your recommendation to try hearing aids. Change any one of these three components of the Habit Loop and you are likely to change a habit. For clinicians, changing the routine by using best practices may be the way to improve overall quality of care.

There is nothing inherently wrong about relying on published guidelines based largely on expert opinion, as it does represent a starting point for the implementation of quality standards within a clinic; however, clinicians should also be aware that they can develop their own best practice standards by collecting data on outcomes and comparing those outcomes to the procedures that were conducted with each patient during the various segments of the patient journey (see Figure 1–1). Other professions have developed their own set of best practices by following this simple four-step formula:

1. Identify the procedures that are thought to lead to the highest outcomes or best results.
2. Once you have a general understanding of what those procedures may be, study how other practices are implementing

these procedures in their clinic and determine if these procedures contribute to the highest outcomes or best results.

3. Standardize the procedures that contribute to higher outcomes or better results.
4. Execute these procedures in your office with every patient.

Since we think utilizing best practices is likely to result in more favorable patient outcomes, let us delve into them. What are some actual best practices you could implement in your own clinic and feel comfortable they are supported by a reasonable amount of scientific evidence? Kochkin et al. (2010) examined 17 aspects of the patient's journey through a hearing health care practice. The authors found that practices that used comprehensive hearing aid fitting protocols tended to have more satisfied patients compared with practices that used a minimal protocol, which typically consisted of five or fewer best practices. This finding is certainly consistent with many of the foundational principles of quality outlined in the previous two chapters, such as Six Sigma and DMAIC. Unfortunately, there is a paucity of similar studies linking hearing aid outcomes to the implementation of a clinical protocol. In the absence of an adequate evi-

---

@CONNECT

Standardized Protocols

If you are looking for a standardized protocol to implement in your clinic, look no further than your national professional organization. The American Academy of Audiology (AAA) and the International Hearing Society (IHS) have published clinical protocols on their respective Web sites.

The AAA's *Guidelines for the Audiological Management of Adult Hearing Impairment* is particularly helpful because it provides a step-by-step evidence-based approach that can be adapted to any audiology clinic. This document can be found at the AAA Web site here: http://www.audiology.org/resources/documentlibrary/Pages/AdultRehabilitation.aspx/

dence base, clinicians must turn to expert opinion as a starting point for developing best practices. Much additional research is needed in this area, and it is hoped that the advent of a relatively low-cost, web-based office management system (e.g., Sycle.net, Blueprint, and AudServ) will make the data collection and analysis process for developing truly evidence-based best practices easier. At this time, however, reality-based practice warrants the use of published best practice standards.

EXAMPLES OF STANDARDIZED PROCEDURES

Kochkin et al. (2010) outlined a "common sense" hearing aid fitting protocol involving nine items:

- Physical evaluation of the ear and review of the patient's medical/audiologic history
- Measurement of the patient's hearing loss using reliable and accurate measurement techniques on calibrated equipment
- A comprehensive hearing aid selection procedure, including the availability of a telecoil
- Assessment of expectations and establishment of realistic patient expectations
- Performance of quality control measures on the devices, such as 2-cc coupler measures compared with recognized standard
- Evaluation and determination of required gain and output using an independently derived prescriptive fitting approach; using probe-microphone measures to verify the integrity of the prescriptive target
- Using the patient's input as well as other measures, such as loudness discomfort levels (LDLs) and acceptable noise levels (ANLs) to fine-tune the devices
- Providing counseling and rehabilitation services, orientation, and instruction on hearing aid use and adjustment to the devices
- Validating the success of the fitting with industry-accepted self-reports of benefit and satisfaction.

For clinicians unfamiliar with best practices who are looking to get started in the implementation process, these nine best practices from Kochkin et al. (2010) would be a good option. Simply require that each of the nine items be conducted with every patient. On the other hand, a more comprehensive approach to best practices might be warranted.

A comprehensive clinical protocol for the audiological management of adult hearing impairment was published by the American Academy of Audiology (AAA) Task Force in 2006. This AAA guideline contained 43 specific recommendations related to assessment, technical aspects of intervention, audiological rehabilitation, and assessment of outcomes. (The entire protocol was published in the September/October 2006 issue of *Audiology Today*.) A systematic evidence-based review was used by the Task Force to create this guideline. Using established evidence-based practice methods, the AAA Task Force determined that less than one-third of the recommendations within their published guidelines were supported by level 1 to 2 evidence, which, you may recall from Chapter 2, is considered the highest quality of evidence in an evidence-based-practice paradigm. Although this indicates that additional high-quality studies are needed in the field of audiology to support the clinical decision-making process, audiologists can be confident that these published guidelines represent current best clinical practices. Since the majority of clinicians work with adults on a routine basis, the 2006 AAA Task Force guidelines are summarized here. Included in this summary are some updates that take into consideration new technology (e.g., wireless streamers and remote microphones) and current fitting trends (e.g., speech mapping):

1. **Auditory assessment.** An assessment of the auditory system includes the following:

   ■ Comprehensive case history.
   ■ Pure-tone, speech, and immittance audiometry.
   ■ Measurement of loudness discomfort level (LDL).
   ■ Quantification of speech intelligibility in background noise in the unaided condition using a standardized speech-in-noise test.
   ■ Otoscopic inspection and cerumen management.

■ Determination of need for treatment/referral to physician or further testing.

■ Counseling of patient, family, and caregivers on the results and recommendations.

■ Assessment of candidacy and motivation for amplification.

■ Determination of medical clearance as defined by the 1977 FDA guidelines.

■ Identification of patient-specific communication needs to determine specific amplification features such as directional microphone, noise reduction, direct audio input, and so forth

■ Completion of an objective measurement of the pre-treatment hearing handicap. Standardized self-reports/questionnaires for this purpose (more details on each of these later in this chapter) include: (a) APHAB, (b) COSI, (c) HHIE, (d) ECHO, (e) GHABP, and (f) IOI-HA.

■ Determination of patient expectations, motivation, assertiveness, manual dexterity, visual acuity, general health, tinnitus condition, occupational demands, and presence of support system. Some tools that can be used for this purpose include: (a) Characteristics of Amplification Tool (COAT) questionnaire, and (b) Modern counseling techniques (outlined later in the chapter).

2. **Hearing aid selection.** The hearing aid selection process will be based on the results from the procedures outlined under item 1 above.

3. **Quality control.** Objective measures of hearing aid performance are to be obtained prior to the fitting using a 2-cc coupler analysis in the hearing aid test (HAT) box. Such an objective assessment could include:

■ Electroacoustic analysis to insure that instruments meet ANSI specifications

■ Electroacoustic analysis to insure that the final programmed settings have been documented

■ Verification of features' functions (objective electroacoustic analysis or information listening) including:
  ■ Directional microphone

- Noise reduction
- Feedback management system
- Frequency lowering
- T-coil
- FM integration
- Paired communication of hearing aids to remote microphones, and so forth
- Wireless streamer functionality
- Verification of fit, venting, color, and type of the devices.

4. **Fitting and verification.** Verification procedures should be based on a validated hearing aid fitting rationale (e.g., NAL-NL2 or DSL i/o v.5) and are expected to yield optimal audibility and comfort of amplified sound for soft, average, and loud sounds.

- In the hearing aid fitting process, a signal, preferably speechlike, must be presented to the hearing aid microphone as it is worn on the patient's ear with a probe microphone present. This result should be compared with a standardized fitting target or goal.
- In the assistive technology fitting process, selections must be justified based on need. Assistive technology can be used to address the following if hearing aids alone are judged inadequate based on need:
    - Face-to-face communication
    - Broadcast and other electronic media
    - Telephone conversation
    - Sensitivity to alerting signals and environmental stimuli.

5. **Hearing aid orientation.** A thorough hearing aid orientation ensures that patients obtain the desired benefits from amplification as easily and efficiently as possible. Hearing aid orientation is complete only when all appropriate information has been provided and the patient/family member/ caregiver is competent to handle the instruments or declines further postfitting care. Orientation should include:

- Care and use instructions
- Insertion and removal of instruments
- Battery replacement

- Telephone-use practice
- Wearing schedule with goals and expectations.

6. **Counseling and follow-up audiologic rehabilitation.** Systematic follow-up provides patients with a comprehensive understanding of the effects of hearing impairment and offers strategies to mitigate those effects. Fundamentally, hearing aid fitting is the beginning of the treatment process. Comprehensive follow-up care provides a structure that moves the patient to ultimate long-term functionality and acceptance. Counseling and rehabilitation strategies should include:

- Anatomy and physiology of the hearing process
- Understanding the audiogram
- Problems associated with understanding speech in noise
- Appropriate/inappropriate communication behaviors
- Communication strategies
- Listening and repair strategies
- Brain exercise strategies
- Ways to control the environment
- Assertive listening training
- Realistic expectations of amplification
- Stress management
- Speech-reading skills
- Community resources.

7. **Assessing outcomes.** After long-term treatment goals have been reached, it is necessary to quantify the impact their treatment strategy has had on overall communication and/or quality-of-life improvement by readministering handicap surveys and/or speech-in-noise tests utilized in the assessment phase outlined above, and comparing the results of these two sets of tests. Only by measuring the outcomes of treatment can audiologists be assured that interventions make a difference and patients have benefited from their care. From a quality perspective, you can think of the auditory assessment as the pretest measures and the outcome measures as the posttest measures. This means that whatever measures you choose to use in the pretest, such as the COSI, APHAB, and so forth, they are re-administered at a designated time post-fitting. The difference in the results between

the pre- and post-measures is the benefit. A thorough overview of outcome measures is provided later in this chapter.

From a quality management standpoint, your behaviors determine your success and ultimately your results. Obviously, a list of best practices does not tell you *how* to do something. For this reason, the following "how to" section is included. It is not intended to be an exhaustive list of procedures to be conducted on all adults with hearing impairments; rather, this section provides some practical guidance and suggestions on critical components of a standardized clinical protocol that can be readily implemented in any clinic. It is hoped that the following section will provide you with a common-sense springboard on which you can systematize best practices for your own clinic.

COLLABORATIVE ASSESSMENT OF COMMUNICATION ABILITY

There is evidence suggesting that the delivery of health care is evolving to a shared-decision-making model (Charles, Gafni, & Whelan, 1997). In the past health care was delivered in a paternalistic fashion. This meant that the practitioner used their skills to diagnose and recommend what the practitioner thought would be best for the patient, with little or no input from the patient. In essence, under the paternalistic delivery model, the practitioner gives the patient, who plays a very passive role in the process, selected information and tries to convince the patient what is best for them. On the other end of the spectrum, largely as a result of the disruptive innovation summarized in Chapter 1, is the informed-decision model. Under the informed-decision model information from the practitioner is transferred directly to the patient, and the patient makes their decision independent of the practitioner. A good example of the informed-decision model in action would be the delivery of hearing aids and services over the Internet. Given the evolving needs of the aging population (recall the Healthy Agers in Chapter 1), a preferred health care delivery model is shared decision making. As the name implies, shared decision making requires the practitioner and patient to collaborate on goals, treatment plans, and possible outcomes.

Shared decision making means that the patient and provider discuss and evaluate treatment options and together build a consensus. As health care delivery evolves with a continued emphasis on quality, a shared-decision-making process would appear to have the most utility. Charles et al. (1997) provide the following five steps of shared decision making:

1. Establish an atmosphere that is conducive to building trust with patients and enables them to feel understood.
2. Elicit patient preferences so that treatment options discussed are compatible with lifestyle and values of the patient.
3. Transfer technical information, risks, and benefits in an unbiased, clear, and simple way.
4. Weigh the pros and cons of various treatment options in a manner that is easily understood by the patient.
5. Share your treatment preferences and affirm the patient's treatment preferences.

The shared-decision model shown in Figure 3–3 forms the foundation for the collaborative assessment of the patient's communication ability. As most of us know, part of a comprehensive prefitting protocol includes the assessment of the patient's communication ability in the unaided condition. Recall Figure 1–1, which shows the six interaction stations between the clinician and patient. Interaction station 4 is the point in which a comprehensive communication-needs analysis is conducted. During this point of the patient journey practitioners are urged to work closely with the patient to target as many listening situations as

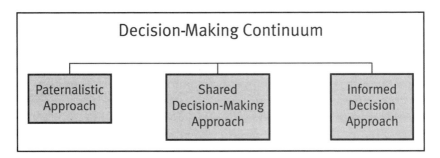

Figure 3–3. A decision-making continuum is shown.

possible for improvement with amplification. Otherwise known as Multiple Environmental Listening Utility (MELU), this means that the hearing health care professional must try to identify ten or more discrete listening situations during the prefitting appointment. Kochkin (2010) has shown that hearing aid users are much more satisfied with their hearing aids depending on the number of listening situations within which their hearing aids have utility. The TELEGRAM is an assessment tool developed by Linda Thibodeaux at the Callier Center in Dallas, Texas (see Figure 1–4 for an example of the TELEGRAM). The TELEGRAM allows the clinician to evaluate more than ten discrete listening situations from a cell phone to meetings, work place listening to alarms in the home. Also notice how there is a space for the clinician to record up to three specific listening situations to target for improvement with amplification; thus, the TELEGRAM is an open-ended needs-assessment tool that can be tailored to the individual. Finally, the TELEGRAM allows the patient and clinician to collaborate on scoring, using a 1 to 5 Likert scale.

There are, of course, several other assessment tools, such as the Client Oriented Scale of Improvement (COSI) from Harvey Dillon and colleagues at the National Acoustic Laboratory in Australia and the Abbreviated Profile of Hearing Aid Benefit (APHAB) from Robyn Cox and colleagues at the University of Memphis that can be used in a manner similar to the TELEGRAM. The main advantage of the TELEGRAM is that is allows both ordinary (e.g., telephone communication) and highly unique and individualized listening situations to be easily recorded and scored. Regardless of the specific needs-assessment tool that you use, take the time to target as many relevant listening situations as possible, and work with the patient to have them rate their ability to hear in the unaided condition for all of them.

Another term that is often used to describe the traditional hearing aid evaluation is "functional communication-needs assessment." Instead of focusing on the product and its features, hearing health care professionals should focus on how to improve listening skills and how to better understand speech in noise. This is the patient's primary complaint which finally brings them into the office, and it is the number one complaint when hearing aids "fail." To address the biggest problem related to hearing aids (speech in noise), we need pretreatment and posttreatment measures (such as QuickSIN and/or HINT) so we can prove to the patient (and ourselves) that we have improved their listening ability in noise. Research from Richard Wilson and colleagues at the VA Medical Center in Mountain Home, Tennessee, indicates that speech-in-noise and speech-in-quiet testing measure different aspects of the auditory system; therefore, both measures need to be included in a standardized prefitting protocol. Since speech-in-quiet testing is usually extensively discussed in introductory textbooks, it is not covered here. On the other hand, since the majority of clinicians fail to conduct speech-in-noise testing, even in the face of good evidence, it warrants some attention in this chapter.

@*CONNECT*

Quality Standards in the United Kingdom

Audiologists Adrian Davis and Pauline Smith of the United Kingdom have written about the use of quality standards in their national health system. They have developed eight quality standards for adults:

- Assessing the service
- Information provision and communication with individuals
- Auditory assessment
- Developing a management plan
- Implementing a management plan
- Outcome
- Professional competence
- Communication and collaborative work.

Using the knowledge gained from Chapters 1 and 2, think about the types of measurement tools you could use to evaluate each one of these standards. These standards may be a good starting point for standardizing quality of care in your practice. See Davis and Smith (2008) for more details on their work.

There are several speech-in-noise tests that can be utilized in the clinic during the prefitting appointment. Although most of them are designed to measure speech intelligibility using sentences, some of them, such as the Acceptable Noise Level test (ANL), do not. If you are looking for one measure of speech intelligibility in noise, the Quick Speech-in-Noise test (QuickSIN) is probably your best bet. The QuickSIN consists of 12 standard equivalent lists, with six sentences in each list (female talker), based on the original IEEE sentences. Five key words in each sentence are scored (i.e., 30 key words for each list). Usually, two lists are presented for each test condition (unaided versus aided). Accompanying the sentences, recorded on the same track, is background four-person babble. The babble becomes 5 dB louder for each subsequent sentence on each list, with SNRs ranging from +25 to 0 dB in 5-dB steps. The test can be scored in percent correct, but typically it is scored in "SNR Loss"—the dB for 50% correct for the patient compared with that of normal-hearing individuals. The pediatric version, BKB-SIN, test uses British children's sentences with male talker. In both cases, four-talker babble is used for the competing noise, and SNR-50 (signal-to-noise ratio for 50% correct key words in sentences) is estimated. The QuickSIN is available from Etymotic Research in Elk Grove Village, Illinois. Here is the step-by-step procedure for conducting the QuickSIN test:

1. Place the earphones on the patient.
2. Zero the VU meter with the calibration tone.
3. Instruct the patient on the required task (see the QuickSIN manual for details).
4. Using a bracketing procedure, identify the patient's most comfortable listening (MCL) level, which is defined as a "loud but okay level of loudness for listening to conversational speech" (item 4 on the well-known IHAFF loudness chart).
5. Familiarize the patient with the procedure by presenting one block of six sentences.
6. Present the sentences at a "loud but okay MCL." This is approximately 70 dB HL.
7. Present the first sentence +25-dB SNR. Note that the CD precalculates the SNR, and you do not need to move the audiometer dials or buttons to change the SNR.
8. Score the number of key words correct.

9. Conduct two runs per ear and calculate SNR loss for each ear by averaging the scores obtained on both runs.
10. Record the SNR loss (25.5 minus the total number of key words correct) for each ear.

Another speech test gaining some popularity over the past few years is the Acceptable Noise Level (ANL) test. Although it has been around for several years, it has been shown in some recent research that it might be a reasonably good predictor of hearing aid satisfaction. The ANL does not measure speech intelligibility; rather, it measures annoyance to sound. It does this by comparing the unaided MCL level with a second measure called the background noise level. The difference between these two measures is referred to as the acceptable noise level.

Perhaps a good way to think about the use of the ANL is as a replacement for traditional MCL testing, which most clinicians learn how to conduct during their training. The ANL test, which can be conducted in just a few minutes, allows you to talk intelligently with the patient about issues related to noise annoyance during the prefitting appointment. That is because annoyance from background noise is such a prevalent problem among hearing aid users that taking the time to measure a potential problem with noise annoyance during the prefitting appointment would seem to be a wise use of time. Recent research on the ANL indicates that the reliability of the test is very sensitive to how the instructions are given to the patient; thus, to ensure good test-retest reliability, clinicians must follow the printed instructions that accompany the test carefully.

Taylor and Bernstein (2011) created the Red Flag Matrix, which is an excellent counseling tool that combines the ANL and QuickSIN test results to quickly provide practical insights about the patient's ability to understand speech in noise and annoyance from noise. The Red Flag Matrix also delineates whether the patient is likely to need advanced technology with noise reduction and/or assistive listening devices (i.e., remote/companion microphones). Quite simply, the QuickSIN and ANL scores are charted on a four-quadrant matrix and this information is used to counsel patients on their possibility of being at risk for lower than expected hearing aid outcomes. Ideas on counseling patients based on charting their scores on the Red Flag Matrix are shown in Figure 3–4. Both the Red Flag Matrix

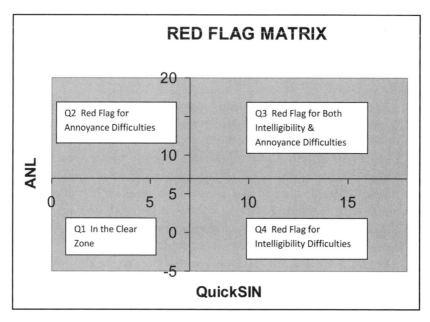

Figure 3–4. A red flag matrix counseling tool is shown. *ANL*, acceptable noise levels; *QuickSIN*, Quick Speech-in-Noise Test.

and TELEGRAM are among the tools that can be used to collect data about patient status prior to the fitting. Form a quality standpoint, the Red Flag Matrix provides you with meaningful patient-centric data.

QUALITY INSPECTION

In addition to data that are collected directly from the patient during the prefitting appointment, it is helpful to evaluate the quality of the ear impression and acoustic coupling system (earmolds). An important data point to be collected during the prefitting is ear-impression quality. This data point, perhaps more than others, is subject to professional bias. (Most clinicians are thought to be relatively poor judges of the quality for their own ear impression.) A common complaint of patients is the physical comfort of their hearing aid fitting. Extraordinary care and attention while taking ear impressions is critically important to avoid postfitting modifications. These modifications, which include grinding earmolds, are certainly an inefficient use of time for professionals and very inconvenient for the patient. Specifically, if the ear mold impression is not meeting the high standards of the clinician, it should likely be redone immediately. Along with a high-quality ear impression, selection of the proper coupling system is essential. It is the responsibility of the professional to carefully evaluate and select the acoustic coupling system that provides optimal comfort while maintaining appropriate gain without feedback. Audiologists cannot rely on automatic feedback presettings to replace their expert judgment of the most appropriate earmold style and material.

ROUTINE USE OF A QUESTIONNAIRE

In a reality-based-practice paradigm, questionnaires can be used to collect and quantify an assortment of information about the patient. Some experts refer to these questionnaires as "income" measurements because they are designed to measure several patient variables before the patient is seen, such as expectations, perceived hearing handicap, and attitude toward receiving help. In addition to gathering information from the patient about expectations, motivation, and self-perception of a hearing problem using a formalized methodology (i.e., 1–5 Likert scale), it is thought that the act of administering a questionnaire adds to the patient's perception of quality and credibility. This is probably due to the fact that the act of conducting a survey has the potential to enhance feelings of trustfulness on the part of the patient because you are asking the patient to provide you with data in a relatively scientific manner.

There are several nonaudiological variables, such as expectations, degree of self-confidence, manual dexterity, and attitude, that contribute to the success of the fitting. Administering a prefitting questionnaire enables you to obtain a more accurate appraisal of many of these nonaudiological variables by measuring them on a scale. There are dozens of prefitting questionnaires that have been developed over the years. As you develop your clinical protocol, it is up to you to decide which variables (expectations, hearing handicap, etc.) you would like to measure with a questionnaire. The following sections represent a sampling of some of the questionnaires that can be used during the prefitting appointment.

Characteristics of Amplification Tool

The Characteristics of Amplification Tool (COAT) was developed by Craig Newman and Sharon Sandridge, two audiologists at Cleveland Clinic, in 2006. The COAT has nine questions that evaluate several important prefitting dimensions, including technology and hearing aid style preferences. The COAT is designed to discover patient preferences and attitudes toward hearing aid use, so that the practitioner can make one firm recommendation at the end of the fitting appointment. The COAT, which is shown in Figure 3–5, can be downloaded and customized by going to http://www.audiologyonline.com and conducting a key word search using the term COAT. (Look for the article published by Sharon Sandridge and Craig Newman of Cleveland Clinic in March 2006.)

Hearing Handicap Inventory for the Elderly—Screening Version

Hearing handicap is best defined as the patient's perception of a problem or limitation in daily communication associated with hearing loss. In order to learn more about a patient's communication handicap, any number of self-assessment tools can be used to measure the degree of the problem. There are several self-assessment tools that can be used to measure hearing handicap. One example of a self-assessment hearing handicap scale that can be used in a busy office is the Hearing Handicap Inventory for the Elderly—Screening Version (HHIE-S) shown in Figure 3–6. This is a 10-question self-report that can be administered to both the patient and a significant other during the prefitting appointment.

Characteristics of Amplification Tool (COAT)

Name: _____ Date: _____

Our goal is to maximize your ability to hear so that you can more easily communicate with others. In order to reach this goal, it is important that we understand your communication needs, your personal preferences, and your expectations. By having a better understanding of your needs, we can use our expertise to recommend the hearing aids that are most appropriate for you. By working together we will find the best solution for you.

Please complete the following questions. Be as honest as possible. Be as precise as possible. Thank you.

1. Please list the top three situations where you would most like to hear better. Be as specific as possible.

    _____

    _____

    _____

2. How important is it for you to hear better? Mark an X on the line.

    Not Very Important   --- *Very Important*

3. How motivated are you to wear and use hearing aids? Mark an X on the line.

    Not Very Motivated   --- *Very Motivated*

4. How well do you think hearing aids will improve your hearing? Mark an X on the line.

    I expect them to:

    Not be helpful   --- *Greatly improve my*
    at all   *hearing*

5. What is your most important consideration regarding hearing aids? Rank order the following factors with 1 as the most important and 4 as the least important. Place an X on the line if the item has no importance to you at all.

    ____ Hearing aid size and the ability of others not to see the hearing aids

    ____ Improved ability to hear and understand speech

    ____ Improved ability to understand speech in noisy situations (e.g., restaurants, parties)

    ____ Cost of the hearing aids

Figure 3–5. Characteristics of Amplification Tool (COAT) is shown. *(continues)*

6. Do you prefer hearing aids that: (check one)

___ are totally automatic so that you do not have to make any adjustments to them.
___ allow you to adjust the volume and change the listening programs as you see fit.
___ no preference

7. Look at the pictures of the hearing aids. Please place an X on the picture or pictures of the style you would NOT be willing to use. Your audiologist will discuss with you if your choices are appropriate for you – given your hearing loss and physical shape of your ear.

BTE

Full Shell

Canal

Mini BTE

Half Shell/ Low profile

CIC

8. How confident do you feel that you will be successful in using hearing aids.

Not Very Confident --*Very Confident*

9. There is a wide range in hearing aid prices. The cost of hearing aids depends on a variety of factors including the sophistication of the circuitry (for example, higher level technology is more expensive than the more basic hearing aids) and size/style (for example, the CIC hearing aids are more expensive than the BTE instruments). The price ranges listed below are for *two* hearing aids. Please check the cost category that represents the maximum amount you are willing to spend. Please understand that you are not locked into that price range. It is just very helpful for us to know your budget so that we can provide you with the most appropriate hearing aids.

___ Basic digital hearing aids: Cost is between $2000 to $2499
___ Basic Plus hearing aids: Cost is between $2500 to $2999
___ Mid-level digital hearing aids: Cost is between $3000 to $3999
___ Premium digital hearing aids: Cost is between $4000 to $6000

Thank you for answering the questions.
Your responses will assist us in providing you with the best hearing healthcare.

Figure 3–5. *(continued)*

HEARING HANDICAP INVENTORY FOR ADULTS - SCREENER

INSTRUCTIONS: The purpose of this questionnaire is to identify the problems your hearing loss may be causing you. Circle Yes, Sometimes, or No for each question. DO NOT SKIP A QUESTION IF YOU AVOID A SITUATION BECAUSE OF A HEARING PROBLEM.

E-1	Does your hearing problem cause you to feel embarrassed when meeting new people?	Yes	Sometimes	No
E-2	Does a hearing problem cause you to feel frustrated when talking to members of your family?	Yes	Sometimes	No
S-1	Does a hearing problem cause you difficulty hearing/understanding co-workers, clients or customers?	Yes	Sometimes	No
E-3	Do you feel handicapped by a hearing problem?	Yes	Sometimes	No
S-2	Does a hearing problem cause you difficulty when visiting friends, relatives or neighbors?	Yes	Sometimes	No
S-3	Does a hearing problem cause you difficulty in the movies or theater?	Yes	Sometimes	No
E-4	Does a hearing problem cause you to have arguments with family members?	Yes	Sometimes	No
S-4	Does a hearing problem cause you difficulty when listening to the TV or radio?	Yes	Sometimes	No
E-5	Do you feel that any difficulty with your hearing limits or hampers your personal or social life?	Yes	Sometimes	No
S-5	Does a hearing problem cause you difficulty when at a restaurant with relatives or friends?	Yes	Sometimes	No

Figure 3–6. Hearing Handicap Inventory for the Elderly is shown. *(continues)*

HEARING HANDICAP INVENTORY FOR ADULTS - SIGNIFICANT OTHER SCREENER

INSTRUCTIONS: The purpose of this questionnaire is to identify the problems your hearing loss may be causing you. Circle Yes, Sometimes, or No for each question. DO NOT SKIP A QUESTION IF YOU AVOID A SITUATION BECAUSE OF A HEARING PROBLEM.

E-1	Does a hearing problem cause your spouse to feel embarrassed when meeting new people?	Yes	Sometimes	No
E-2	Does a hearing problem cause your spouse to feel frustrated when talking to members of your family?	Yes	Sometimes	No
S-1	Does a hearing problem cause your spouse difficulty hearing/understanding co-workers, clients or customers?	Yes	Sometimes	No
E-3	Does your spouse feel handicapped by a hearing problem?	Yes	Sometimes	No
S-2	Does a hearing problem cause your spouse difficulty when visiting friends, relatives or neighbors?	Yes	Sometimes	No
S-3	Does a hearing problem cause your spouse difficulty in the movies or theater?	Yes	Sometimes	No
E-4	Does a hearing problem cause your spouse to have arguments with family members?	Yes	Sometimes	No
S-4	Does a hearing problem cause your spouse difficulty when listening to the TV or radio?	Yes	Sometimes	No
E-5	Do you feel that any difficulty with hearing limits or hampers your spouse's personal or social life?	Yes	Sometimes	No
S-5	Does a hearing problem cause your spouse difficulty when at a restaurant with relatives or friends?	Yes	Sometimes	No

Figure 3–6. *(continued)*

The HHIE-S allows the patient to evaluate the emotional and social impact their hearing loss has on communication. The HHIE-S is scored by having the patient answer "yes," "sometimes," or "no" to 10 questions. Four points are assigned if the patient answers "yes," two points are assigned if the patient answers "sometimes," and 0 points are awarded if the patient answers "no" to any of the questions. The point totals are calculated and a degree of handicap is determined using the published norms.

The score from the HHIE-S helps determine the patient's perception of hearing handicap and, to some extent, their motivation to receive services from your office. As mentioned previously, an added benefit of the HHIE-S is that it can be administered to both the patient and a companion. Valuable insights about motivation can be obtained when scores for both people are compared. For example, if the patient has a low score of 4 (no perception of the problem) and their companion has a higher score of 24 (moderate perception of problem), this is an indication that the patient is denying a hearing loss or has no motivation for receiving help.

Of course, there are several other aspects of patient status that can be evaluated with questionnaires. For example, expectations can be evaluated using the Expected Consequences of Hearing Aid Ownership (ECHO) developed by Robyn Cox. Reality-based practice requires clinicians to identify one or two components of communication status and begin measuring them with a questionnaire.

Let us turn our attention to another often overlooked best practice, which is prefitting counseling techniques.

CONTEMPORARY COUNSELING TECHNIQUES

Beck and Harvey (2009) recommend the routine use of cognitive behavioral therapy and motivational interviewing as techniques that help patients uncover the emotional impact of their hearing loss with the guidance of the clinician. These techniques should be used to help the patient internalize and express their needs, desires, and motivation for amplification. It is important to realize there are essentially no studies in the professional literature that endorse the way most professionals counsel (explaining the audiogram, talking about hearing aid features, and making the hearing aids a commodity); therefore, modern counseling techniques, namely motivational interviewing, is a strategy for improving the overall quality of the interaction between the clinician and the patient.

Harvey (2001) outlines the process of circular questioning, which is a specific motivational interviewing technique. Here is an example of circular questioning that may occur during the prefitting appointment:

- Who referred you and who knows about your appointment?
- Who is most concerned about your possible hearing loss? Second most? Third most?
- Which of the above persons would be most concerned if you did or did not get hearing aids? Second most? Third most?
- Given that you get/not get hearing aids, what would (person X, Y, Z) say or do to each other? How might that help or hinder you?
- Then what would (person X, Y, Z) do with you? Then what would you do with them? How would that affect you?

The use of circular questioning helps the clinician uncover the "cast of characters" involved in the communication challenges of the patient; thus, the clinician has more insight into the family dynamics the patient faces every day due to their hearing impairment. According to Miller and Rollnick (2002) the audiologist uses techniques from motivational interviewing to elicit four categories of self-motivational statements. This is also called "change talk." Here are some examples of questions you can use surrounding the "change talk" concept:

1. Problem recognition
   - Why did you believe you had a hearing loss prior to coming here?
   - What difficulties have you had in relation to your hearing loss?
   - In what ways do you think you or other people have been affected by your hearing loss?

- How has your hearing loss stopped you from doing what you want to do?

2. Concern

   - What worries you about your hearing loss? What can you imagine happening to you?
   - How do you feel about your hearing loss?
   - How much does that concern you?
   - What do you think will happen if you do not get hearing aids?

3. Stated intention to change

   - What makes you think that you may need to get hearing aids?
   - If you were 100% successful and things worked out exactly as you would like, what would be different?
   - Do you remember a time when your hearing was better? What has changed?
   - How has your hearing loss stopped you from moving forward, from doing what is most important in your life?

4. Degree of self-efficacy to change

   - What encourages you that you can get hearing aids if you want?
   - What might stand in your way of getting hearing aids?
   - What are the options for you now? What could you do?
   - What would be the best results you could imagine if you got hearing aids?

The use of contemporary counseling techniques is an integral part of better understanding the emotional impact and effect on family dynamics that hearing loss of adult onset may have on the individual. This section is merely the tip of the iceberg and is certainly not intended to replace a comprehensive course on the subject of motivational interviewing. Clinicians are encouraged to enroll in a motivational interviewing course to learn more about how these techniques can be implemented in your clinic's best practice protocol.

@*CONNECT*

Neil and Susan Clutterbuck, Quality Mavens

Neil and Susan are the owners of EARtrak, a patient satisfaction tool. This is what they say about quality:

"Our private audiology clinic in Australia regularly receives a report from EARtrak (see http://www.EARtrak.com). The report compares our clients' satisfaction against the benchmarks set by other clinics using the EARtrak system. Major areas of comparison are satisfaction in a wide variety of listening situations, satisfaction with features of the hearing aids (battery usage, comfort, etc.), and satisfaction with the service offered by our clinic.

We use the report to examine what we are doing well, and what we do poorly. We also do comparisons within the clinic—between clinicians, and between hearing aid makes and models. As an example, if my way of fitting hearing aids leaves clients dissatisfied with telephone use, but the evidence shows that Susan's clients are doing well in this area, of course I ask her to help me.

This practice-based evidence is highly relevant—it is about our population of clients, and our range of hearing aid suppliers. The benchmarks are set by our peers using today's technology. If we are falling behind, we need to be aware of that, and make improvements—fast.

Our chase for excellence has allowed us to significantly increase word-of-mouth referrals, and to discontinue paid marketing."

QUALITY CONTROL WITH 2-CC COUPLER MEASURES

Manufacturers rely on 2-cc coupler measures during the quality control process because they are standardized. Every hearing aid they make can be tested using the same cavity that allows the device to be compared with a published standard. As we mentioned previously, there can be some pretty big differences, however, between the hearing aid response in a 2-cc coupler and an actual human ear. Using average data, we can make some reasonable predictions about the differences between the gain obtained in 2-cc coupler and in real ears. This is referred to as the COupler Response for Flat Insertion Gain (CORFIG).

Another critical component of quality control related to the 2-cc coupler is the hearing aid specification sheet, or simply, "the spec sheet." No matter what type or style of hearing aid is being fitted, a spec sheet is required to be sent with the hearing aid by the manufacturer. The American National Standards Institute (ANSI) determines the data that must be reported on the spec sheet. The ANSI S3.22 1996 standards are what are currently used. (There is another similar standard in Europe called IEC.) The 1996 standard has been revised, which is now the S3.22-2003. Using the 2-cc coupler, clinicians can cross-check these measures by ensuring the measures they conduct in their office approximate those listed on the "spec sheet."

VERIFICATION OF PRESCRIPTIVE FITTING METHODS

The functionality of basic and advanced features should be verified in the patient's ear using probe-microphone measures. The use of probe-microphone measures, however, implies that the clinician has a good understanding of the rationale of prescriptive fitting methods. This section implies that clinicians have a good understanding of the rationale of the prescriptive fitting method.

It would be nice, and would save a lot of time, if we could just assume that prescriptive fitting methods, displayed as "simulated gain" on a fitting screen, translated into an accurate match of the prescriptive target in ear canal SPL. Unfortunately, what we see in the 2-cc coupler and on our computer fitting screens usually is not what is actually happening in the real ear. Probe-microphone measures are the gold standard when it comes to verifying that our prescriptive fitting method of choice is being met in the patient's ear canal. There really is no substitute method, and failure to assess the real-ear SPL when hearing aids are fitted is considered unethical practice by many audiologists.

#DISCOVER

More About Prescriptive Fittings

Here are some things to remember about the "first fit" of gain and output:

■ The manufacturer's software will do "first fit," but it is your responsibility to do "last fit."
■ Just because you select a given validated prescription (e.g., NAL-NL2) in the fitting software, this does not assure that you will meet this target in the real ear (in fact, research suggests that you often will not even be within 10 dB of target).
■ Just because a given program appears to meet targets in the simulated fitting screen, this does not mean that you will meet these targets in the real ear.
■ Most manufacturers' proprietary fitting algorithms are geared toward "initial acceptance"; this is different from the validated prescriptive methods, which tend to be geared toward speech intelligibility and preferred loudness levels.
■ Probe-microphone measures must be used to verify the quality of the match to an independently derived prescriptive target.

Probe-microphone measures have been around for a number of decades; however, for reasons that are not clearly understood, not every clinician takes the time to do them. They are, however, absolutely necessary if you want to be sure your prescriptive fitting target is being matched, and are considered "best practice." Any savvy consumer would expect this procedure to be conducted—especially since the topic was addressed thoroughly in a 2009 *Consumer's Report*. After all, if one is purchasing a state-of-the-art electronic device for several thousand dollars, it is only logical that the programming be verified using a state-of-the- art device also. No matter what you might hear from others, there is no way to know if patients are getting the right amount of gain or output without conducting some probe-microphone measures. In essence, they ensure that your patient is starting off with a reasonable good "first fit"—and at the least, reasonable audibility.

Below are some common things to remember when conducting probe-microphone measures for the purpose of verifying the "closeness" of a prescriptive fitting. There are two important things to remember when starting to conduct probe-microphone measures: (1) get the patient in the right position, and (2) get the probe tube in the right place. If you get these two things right, you have a good chance of obtaining a valid and reliable measure.

Positioning the patient is important. Probably the biggest mistake dispensers make is allowing the patient to sit too far away from the loudspeaker. Two reasons why you want to have the patient sit reasonably close (around 1 m) are:

- It will improve the SNR. Often, test rooms are noisy (more than one computer running, heating or air conditioning, etc.). If you want to test at soft levels, such as 50 dB SPL (and you should), then you will have to have the patient at a distance where 50 dB SPL is louder than the ambient noise reaching the monitor microphone; this allows for proper leveling/calibration.
- It will prevent overdriving of the loudspeaker. The farther the person is away from the loudspeaker, the more output required to reach a given desired level. In some cases, with some equipment, you will overdrive the loudspeaker (the run will be aborted) if the person is too far away.

A commonly used method to assure that the patient's head is located at the correct distance is to use a "calibrated string" 1 m long. Tape one end of the string to the top of the loudspeaker, and then assure that the middle of the patient's head is at the other end of the string. It also is important to have the person sit at the correct azimuth. Unless your equipment requires something different (e.g., Fonix 7000), a 0° vertical azimuth and a 0° horizontal azimuth is recommended.

All systems use a probe tube, although the tubes are slightly different among manufacturers. Most systems require that you first "calibrate the tube" (follow the instructions in the manual). This procedure makes the probe tube acoustically invisible; it is as if the microphone itself were located in the ear canal. At the time of testing, you now will place this tube in the patient's ear canal. Poor placement of the probe tube easily can make the entire probe-microphone measure invalid. A few things to remember about placing the probe tube in the ear canal are as follows:

- The tip of the tube needs to be relatively close to the tympanic membrane (TM). If the tip is within 5 mm, valid results should be obtained through 4000 Hz.
- The tip of the tube should be 3 to 5 mm beyond the tip of the hearing aid or earmold.
- The average adult ear canal is about 25 mm. The best reference for probe-tube placement is the intertragal notch. Although it varies from person to person, this notch usually is about 10 mm from the opening of the ear canal. The average distance, therefore, between the tragal notch and the TM is about 35 mm.
- If a marker (or black mark using a Sharpie) is placed on the tube at 30 mm from the tip, and this mark is aligned with the intertragal notch, then the tip of the probe tube should be about 5 mm from the TM. This would satisfy both requirements of being close to the TM and extending beyond the tip of the hearing aid or earmold. As the tip of the probe is farther from the TM, the output in the high frequencies is reduced. If you were not aware of the poor probe placement, this inaccurate finding might prompt you to unnecessarily add high frequencies when the hearing aid is programmed.
- While it is tempting to slide the probe tube through the vent of the hearing aid, do not do this if the vent is 2 mm or smaller, as you will alter the vent effects that you are attempting to measure.

The input signal can be real speech, modulated noise, or unmodulated noise, depending on what equipment you have and what you are assessing. For checking the Maximum Power Output (MPO) of the hearing aid, you also may want to use a swept pure tone (i.e., a tone will drive the hearing aid to a higher output than a broadband signal). You will present the test signals at different input levels; again, the actual levels will depend on what you are measuring. Common presentation levels are 50, 65, and 80 dB SPL for soft, average, and loud, and a swept tone of 85 or 90 dB SPL for the MPO assessment.

There are different input signals available for probe-microphone testing. These signals vary depending on the equipment that you are using and the purpose of the test. Currently, most audiologists use some type of speech signal. In the past, either pure tones or noise for probe-microphone testing have been used, and there still are some cases when you will want to use one of these inputs:

- Swept pure tones: Recommended to determine the MPO of the hearing aid, but a poor choice for other probe-microphone measures. Using a pure-tone signal it is difficult to observe compression and channel interaction effects.
- Broadband noise: A commonly used noise for conducted real-ear insertion gain REIG (e.g., pink noise, speech-shaped noise) but not recommended for real-ear aided response (REAR) verification. Good signal for assessing the effects of digital noise reduction (DNR).

In the past few years, it has become common to use the real-ear aided response (REAR) for verification and a calibrated speech signal as the input. This is now commonly referred to as "speech mapping," a term that was originally coined by Bill Cole of Audioscan in the 1990s. It is also possible to use "live speech," that is, the dispenser (or a family member) can provide the input signal live. Live speech might be helpful for demonstrations, and perhaps adding a little "show" to the fitting, but we do not recommend it for target matching, as fitting targets need to correspond to a given input signal to be accurate.

There are many advantages to the (REAR)/speech mapping SPL-O-Gram approach of fitting hearing aids:

- The graph is more logical—big numbers on the top, small numbers on the bottom.
- The relationship between the patient's hearing loss, fitting targets, and hearing aid output are displayed logically, facilitating counseling.

- The display of both the audiogram and the amplified speech output in ear canal SPL facilitates verification of speech audibility.

- The use of real speech allows for evaluating the hearing aid in its normal-use condition, including effects of multiple channels and advanced signal processing.

- The use of real speech clearly illustrates the effects of wide dynamic range compression, including visualization of effective ratios and influence of time constants.

- The SPL-O-Gram mode is effective for assessing and displaying directional and DNR function.

- The use of real speech adds face validity to the overall fitting process. It is easy for most patients and their significant others to see how hearing aids process live speech on the probe mic's display monitor.

At the time of the fitting, using either the REIG or REAR/ speech mapping, the general goal is to "match" the target. How close of a match is necessary? In general, it is suggested that you attempt to have a match within ±5 dB of the fitting target, at least through the frequencies of 3000 Hz. Also, attempt to follow the general slope of the fitting target, that is, you would not want to be 5 dB over target at 1500 Hz and 5 dB below target at 2000 Hz.

In particular, it is useful to observe the target for soft speech, and not fall too far below this mark, as one of the primary benefits the patient will obtain is audibility for soft sounds (although they might not thank you for it for several weeks). Recognize, of course, that these targets are only a "starting point." Research has shown that about 60% of patients have preferred gain within ±3 dB of the target for average inputs. This means that nearly 50% of patients will have preferred gain levels that are significantly higher or lower—but you have to start somewhere. One recent study by Abrams, Chisolm, McManus, and McArdle (2012) compared a manufacturer's "first fit" setting with a verified match of a prescription target (NAL-NL1). Using the APHAB as an outcome, results indicated most patients not only preferred the settings of the verified match of a prescription target, but the majority of patients derived more benefit from it as well.

Typically, probe-microphone measures are conducted during the hearing aid fitting appointment. A basic verification measure that evaluates how close the fitting is to a prescriptive target takes about 5 to 10 minutes, and since it is an objective measure probe-microphone measures are considered an essential part of standardization of the clinical process.

Let us now turn our attention to what clinicians can do to enhance quality during the hearing aid fitting appointment.

HEARING AID ORIENTATION

Research has shown that when you spend quality time with your patients, methodically orienting and instructing them on the use, care, and expectations of their hearing aids, overall patient satisfaction is high. Here are three easy-to-follow steps of a well-executed hearing aid orientation process:

1. Use

   - Instruct the patient on insertion and removal of the devices. Have them attempt to conduct this task in your office in front of you. You will have to show the patient how to hold the hearing aids during the insertion process (conduct this training over something "soft," as the hearing aids *will be* dropped). You will have to instruct them on adjusting the volume control, the remote, and any additional switches the hearing aids may have. Additionally, you need to demonstrate to the patient how to use the telephone with their new hearing aids. It is important to create a real-world situation, for example, they answer a ringing telephone.
   - Instruct the patient on care and maintenance. The patient needs to be shown how to clean the hearing aid. This involves showing the patient how cerumen is removed from the end of the hearing aid. Part of care and maintenance is also instructing the patient on how to change the battery and how to store the instruments when they are not being worn.

2. Expectations

   - If you are fitting a new hearing aid user, you will want to be sure to place him on a wearing schedule. A wearing schedule allows the patient to become acclimated to new sounds they are hearing. As a rule of thumb, new hearing aid users should start wearing their hearing aids at home in a relaxed and quiet situation for a few days before wearing them in more demanding listening situations, such as a restaurant. There is no reason the average new user needs more than a week to begin full-time use. The bottom line is that the patients need to give themselves a few days to get up to speed with their new devices, going from relatively easy to more difficult listening situations.

3. Offering Reassurance

■ Most of us know there are several potential negative emotions surrounding hearing loss. Many of these emotions are still present on the day of the fitting. It is important to be patient and offer support for each individual, especially during their initial foray with hearing aids. No matter how frustrated you may feel regarding those patients who are "just not getting it," you need to remain patient.

One tactic that you can use to ensure your patients are adjusting to their new hearing aids is to phone them a day or two after the initial fitting. This small gesture is an excellent way to uncover any problems, for example, is the patient having trouble inserting the hearing aids into their ears? At the same time, it sends positive messages to each patient by showing them that you care, and that you are going the extra mile to serve them.

Before you send the patient home with their new hearing aids, it is helpful to review a simple checklist with them. This will ensure that you have covered all the main points that often cause confusion or unnecessary stress for the patient. In case you might think that you have already told the patient what they need to know, here are some data about informational counseling, provided by University of Minnesota audiologist Bob Margolis:

■ Only about 50% of the information provided by health care providers is retained; depending on conditions, 40 to 80% may be forgotten immediately.

■ Of the information that patients do recall, they remember about half *incorrectly*. So half is forgotten immediately, and half of what is remembered is wrong. Consider that

---

#DISCOVER

Hearing Aid Checklist

Using the best practice guidelines outlined in this chapter, it is up to you to develop and implement your own standardized protocol. A checklist like this can be used to ensure that the standardized protocol is completed at the time of the hearing aid fitting appointment:

■ Verified prescriptive match of gain/output target (±5 dB) using probe-microphone measures
■ Assured that loud sounds were not uncomfortably loud
■ Assured that patient found the quality of the programmed gain and output "acceptable"
■ No acoustic feedback in typical use conditions
■ Hearing aids fit properly (not too loose or too tight)
■ Instructed on insertion and removal of hearing aids, and patient can now put hearing aids in and take them out
■ Demonstrated how to use hearing aids with telephones
■ Instructed on proper use of volume control and/or remote control
■ Counseled on initial use of the hearing aids and realistic expectations (reviewed wearing schedule for the first week to 10 days)
■ Instructed on care, cleaning, proper storage, and batteries
■ Gave phone number to call with questions or problems
■ Approximately 1 hour of face-to-face time spent with the patient

if you remove 50% of the facts you told the patient about their hearing loss and hearing aids, and then distort half the remaining information, the result could be a highly misunderstood message.

■ Patients often forget their medical diagnoses. One study reported that patients could not recall 68% of the diagnoses told to them in a medical visit. When there were multiple diagnoses, patients could not recall the most important diagnosis 54% of the time. Another study found that after counseling, patients and the health care provider agreed on problems that required follow-up only 45% of the time.

These disturbing data about informational counseling certainly point out the importance of including information for the patient to take home. A hearing aid checklist is a good starting point.

AUDITORY TRAINING AND AURAL REHABILITATION

The final best practice worth careful consideration is follow-up care. This is sometimes referred to as aftercare or aural rehabilitation. In general, aftercare is anything clinicians do with the patient following the fitting of hearing aids. Aftercare can be conducted on an individual basis with each patient or aftercare can be provided to small groups. The reality is that the majority of clinicians fail to conduct aftercare even in the face of data (e.g., Northern & Beyer, 1999) suggesting otherwise. Aural rehabilitation is a service every clinician should provide to patients.

In addition to reducing return for credit rates, aftercare is an essential part of the services clinicians deliver to patients. Today, as patients have gained more access to information through the Internet and other sources, they have come to realize there are supplemental exercises available to them that will help them improve their listening skills. Additionally, better educated patients seeking these types of services tend to be more demanding, and are willing to shop around for this service until they find it. For the clinician this means he or she must be ready to incorporate new and innovative tools into their practice if they want to remain competitive.

Although aural rehabilitation programs have failed to be widely embraced by the profession and patients alike, recently published reports indicate that the winds of change may be blowing. Patients are also being encouraged to think beyond the device as a solution for their communication deficits. In a recently published open letter to patients they were urged to fully participate in the rehabilitation process if they want to get their money's worth from their investment of new hearing aids. There also have been recent articles published in trade journals touting the overall effectiveness that self-guided aural rehabilitation programs have on lowering returns for credit, something that has plagued the industry for decades.

To this point, the terms "aural rehabilitation" and "auditory training" have been used synonymously. It is important to point out the difference between these two terms. For our purposes, aural rehabilitation is a much broader term encompassing several aspects of nonmedical treatment for hearing loss. Traditionally, aural rehabilitation is offered to patients as a supplemental service when hearing aids are acquired. For example, aural rehabilitation could be general counseling, basic education about the ear and hearing, speech-reading classes, assertive training, hearing aid orientation groups, or formal instruction on communication skills.

On the other hand, auditory training relates to a much narrower view of therapy. Auditory training relates to exercises patients can do to improve listening and communication, the focus of which is on improving various components of auditory memory and comprehension. Auditory training is thought to take advantage of the neuroplasticity of the auditory system. Even though there is some evidence supporting its effectiveness, auditory training has been thought to be both repetitive and dull. Recently, however, computer-based self-guided tools have been introduced commercially. These training tools are more "high tech" and are thought to be more engaging for the patient, which is likely to result in increased use of the training exercises. There is also some evidence that auditory exercises are not effective with all patients. In a three-site randomized control trials with 263 veterans comparing LACE auditory training to informational counseling and a placebo (non-focused interaction with the clinician) she found all four groups experienced small, but significant improvements in handicap reduction and hearing aid benefit. Thus, auditory training did not outperform other types of follow-up services. Additionally, Saunders (2012) did find that a small number of individuals did significantly benefit from LACE auditory training (a commercially available type of auditory training available from Neurotone). These results suggest that audiologists need to collaborate with patients in customizing the appropriate type of auditory training and aural rehabilitation.

If we focus only on computer-assisted auditory training programs for adults, there are five programs available clinically. All of them are designed to take advantage of the plasticity of the auditory system. Additionally, there are several anecdotal reports and a couple of studies from nonrefereed publications showing that the consistent use of an auditory training program can lower returns for credit.

Although lower returns for credit do not necessarily equate to improved patient satisfaction, all of us can agree that lower returns are desirable. Considering the clinical evidence of effectiveness for auditory training and its underutilization in most practices, it is obvious that the majority of audiologists are overlooking the value of computer-based auditory training programs such as the following:

1. Computer-Assisted Speech Perception Testing and Training at the Sentence Level (CASPERSent). CASPERSent is a multimedia program designed by Arthur Boothroyd. The primary training target is perceptual skill. The program consists of 60 sets of City University of New York (CUNY) sentences representing 12 topics and three sentence types. Sentences are presented by lipreading only, hearing only, and a combination of the two. Patients are required to hear and/or see a spoken sentence, repeat as much as possible, view the text, click on the words correctly identified, see/hear the sentence again, and move on to the next sentence. The CASPERSent can be self-administered or administered with the aid of another person. For more information visit http://www.rohan.sdsu.edu/~aboothro/files/CASPERSENT/CasperSent_preprint.pdf/.

2. Computer-Assisted Tracking Simulation and Computer-Assisted Speech Training (CATS). The CATS program, which was developed at the Central Institute for the Deaf in St. Louis and subsequently updated by Harry Levitt, allows the patient and another person to interact. It works the following way: The talker says a sentence or phrase, and the listener repeats verbatim the sentence or phrase. If the sentence is correct, the talker goes on to another sentence or phrase. If it is incorrect, the talker repeats some variation of the utterance until the listener correctly repeats it. The computer-based tracking program makes it easier to score the results of each session and monitor progress.

3. Computer-Assisted Speech Training (CAST). Like the previously mentioned auditory training programs, CAST was originally designed for adults with cochlear implants, but, like the other two, it can be adapted for use with adult hearing aid wearers. CAST uses more than 1,000 novel words spoken by four different talkers. The CAST program is adaptive in that the level of difficulty is automatically adjusted according to the patient's performance. To learn more about CAST, visit http://www.tigerspeech.com/tst_cast.html/.

4. Listening and Communication Enhancement (LACE). The LACE program is a user-friendly, computer-based program for both patients and clinicians. Patients are required to complete a series of short exercises that are intended to boost their auditory memory and speed of processing. LACE can be completed on any home computer and results can be tabulated and shared with the clinician using the Internet. Recently, Neurotone, the creators of LACE, introduced both a DVD and an on-line version to make it even more accessible. LACE was originally designed to be completed at home by the patient; however, many clinics around the country are seeing increased patient compliance when at least some of the exercises are completed in the clinic. For more information visit http://www.neurotone.com/.

Historically, auditory training programs have been viewed by some as largely academic exercises that are conducted in a university clinic. With the evolution of computer technology and the Internet over the past decade or so, audiologists need to reconsider the use of computer-based auditory training. Although an array of questions remain unresolved (e.g., which program is most effective for different adult populations), there is evidence supporting the efficacy of computer-based auditory training programs. Given the relatively steady in-the-drawer and return for credit rates plaguing our industry, it is imperative that professionals embrace computer-based auditory training programs. Without a doubt, computer-based auditory training needs to be part of a more comprehensive aural rehabilitation program that we offer our patients.

#DISCOVER

Intangible Aspects of Clinical Quality

This chapter lists several tangible aspects of clinical quality. These are aspects of quality that can be measured in an objective manner. On the other hand, there are several intangible aspects of quality that cannot be directly measured but are nonetheless very important. Your personal appearance and the appearance of your office are two intangible aspects of quality that cannot be overlooked. Believe it or not, wearing a lab coat enhances your perceived professionalism. This is a good example of an intangible aspect of quality.

DATA-DRIVEN RESULTS

Thus far we have discussed best practices to be employed in the hearing aid selection and fitting process. Given that a significant part of quality in the clinic is systematically measuring the actual results of the fitting, let us turn our attention to outcome measures. Hearing aid outcome measures are really designed to answer one important question for the patient: "How much have I solved your problem since we started working together?"

Fortunately, there are several tools at our disposal to help us answer this question. The current state of outcome measures seems to be an informal assessment of results following the fitting. Worse yet, quality oftentimes is judged solely on the patient *not* returning the hearing aids for credit. As you know by now, that is a completely inadequate method for evaluating quality. Sadly, according to Humes (2012) just 36% of audiologists routinely use self-reports of outcomes. This low percentage may reflect the fact that audiologists do not see the value of outcome measures. Another possible reason related to their lack of implementation is the sheer number of questionnaires available. Given the number of self-report questionnaires that measure a myriad of different dimensions of outcome, the purpose of this section is to demystify the rationale of hearing aid outcome measures. After reading this section you will better understand the various dimensions of outcome, methods of measuring outcomes, data that support the use of different outcome measures, and, finally, how the routine use of outcome measures is an essential component of any quality initiative.

In technical terms, an outcome measure quantifies the overall effectiveness of your intervention or treatment plan. In practical terms, outcome measures more or less provide you and the patient results of their investment in hearing aids. There are several dimensions or domains of hearing aid outcome that can be evaluated, and one of the challenges is to not get bogged down in all the different dimensions. They include the following:

- Daily use
- Sound quality
- Speech understanding
- Loudness normalization
- Listening effort
- Quality of life
- Social interaction
- Reduced burden of significant other.

The first thing you should notice about this list is that some of the dimensions are directly related to the performance of the hearing aids. For example, sound quality, speech understanding, and loudness normalization are directly related to the quality of the product and how it is programmed. These are commonly referred to as device components of hearing aid outcomes. On the other hand, there are other dimensions of outcome that measure the impact the hearing aids have on issues related to improving the hearing handicap which often results from the hearing loss. Domains such as social interaction, quality of life, and reduced burden on significant others are examples of these nondevice components. Indirectly, of course, they could be device related; for example, if the hearing aids were not programmed correctly, it is very unlikely that quality of life will improve.

BENEFIT VERSUS SATISFACTION: WHAT YOU ARE MEASURING

The difference between a patient's unaided performance and aided performance is called benefit. Any time we administer a test in the unaided condition and compare it with the aided condition we are measuring benefit. Hearing aid benefit can be defined as the difference between unaided and aided performance measured either objectively or subjectively.

Hearing aid benefit can be measured objectively by comparing aided and unaided measures of speech recognition ability; for example: a patient's QuickSIN SNR loss improved by 5 dB when they were aided. Hearing aid benefit also can be measured subjectively through the use of self-report measures, commonly called questionnaires; for example: a person had 70% problems in background noise without hearing aids, and only 30% of problems using amplification.

Because objective tests are usually completed using a predefined external standard, they are almost exclusively tests that take place in the laboratory (research studies), clinic, or office. While this type of testing can provide meaningful results, the test environment often does not reflect the actual-use conditions for the patient; therefore, self-report measures of outcome are a useful method of determining real-world benefits of hearing aid performance.

#*DISCOVER*

Outcome Terminology

The World Health Organization has classified various domains of outcome in the following way (each domain can be assessed with a different outcome measure):

Disorder: Occurs as a result of some type of disease process or malformation of the auditory system (e.g., presbycusis)

Impairment: Any loss or abnormality of psychological, physiologic, or anatomic structure or function (e.g., high-frequency hearing loss)

Disability: Any restriction or lack of ability to perform an activity in the manner or within the range considered normal (e.g., unable to understand average speech-in-background noise)

Handicap: A disadvantage for a given individual, resulting from an impairment or a disability, that limits or prevents the fulfillment of a role that is normal, based on their age, gender, as well as social and cultural factors (e.g., unable to continue coaching basketball because of speech-in-noise understanding problems)

Activity Limitations: Difficulties an individual may have in executing activities (e.g., unable to understand television when there is background noise)

Participation Restrictions: Problems an individual might experience in individual life situations (e.g., avoids gathering with friends at neighborhood tavern to watch football on TV)

Audiologists are encouraged to find self-reports that address these various dimensions of outcome, many of which are reviewed in this text.

Another separate dimension of a hearing aid fitting outcome is satisfaction. Satisfaction differs from benefit in that satisfaction is not necessarily performance driven. For example, a patient can have a significant degree of benefit as measured on any aided and unaided tests, but they might be reporting dissatisfaction as measured on a satisfaction scale. Most hearing care professionals would agree that satisfaction is a nebulous dimension of outcome because it comprises many variables, such as professionalism of the staff, cleanliness of the office, and wait time in the reception area. Satisfaction is also highly correlated to expectations—to state the obvious, people who have fairly low expectations are the easiest to satisfy. People who receive free hearing aids tend to be more satisfied, although the difference is not as much as you might think. Even though satisfaction does comprise many dimensions, just like benefit, it can be measured using a questionnaire.

CLINIC VERSUS REAL WORLD: HOW TO MEASURE OUTCOME

There are two different ways we can measure hearing aid outcomes. The first way is using a laboratory or clinical measure. These measures consist of any type of measurement you would conduct in your office or clinic, typically in the test booth. As a general rule, laboratory measures are objective in nature and engage the patient in some type of quantifiable task. This means the patient is required to complete some type of test, and results are scored as the percent correct (or incorrect) and compared with normative data. The objective nature of laboratory tests makes them valuable because you can quickly compare scores to an average. Additionally, the test can be specifically designed to collect important information regarding the functioning of the hearing aids (e.g., Does the directional microphone technology improve speech understanding when there is a talker in front and noise originates from behind?). The downside to laboratory tests is that they often are conducted in contrived listening environments that are not reflective of everyday listening conditions; or the listening task itself is something that the listener will rarely experience.

Although they are considered subjective in nature, self-assessment inventories or questionnaires of hearing aid outcome capture patients' judgments of hearing aid benefit and satisfaction in real-world listening conditions. For this reason, self-reports of outcome are usually considered to be the gold standard when it comes to measuring hearing aid outcomes because they capture success (or lack thereof) in everyday listening places; however, there are a couple of pitfalls associated with self reports. First, if the questionnaire does not capture situations the individual patient is familiar with, the information you are gathering is essentially meaningless because the measure does not reflect that patient's daily experience. A second issue is that the questionnaire may not be specific enough, for example, general questions about understanding in background noise might not reveal the benefit of directional microphone technology, even though lab findings show that the algorithm is working effectively. A final drawback is associated with variability. The way you administer (hand it to the patient or mail it to them), the personality of the patient (do they want to please you?), and even when you administer it (the day of the fitting or 6 months after) all potentially effect the results. Do not, however, equate those pitfalls with a lack of validity. Self-reports, when properly standardized and validated, are accurate and reflective of the patient's experiences. Your job is simply to choose the best self-report for the patients you typically see on a daily basis. What self-assessment inventory answers the questions about which you are most concerned?

LABORATORY MEASURES OF OUTCOME

Let us turn our attention to the laboratory or clinical measures of hearing aid outcome. These outcome measures often are conducted on the day of the fitting, although testing at follow-up visits also can provide useful information. There are a wide array of laboratory measures of outcome we could use. Many of them, however, are not useful clinically because they are time-consuming, or because the results of the laboratory measure do not relate directly to patient counseling. The procedures outlined below are intended to provide you with a general idea of how much benefit the patient may be experiencing at any given point in time following the fitting. Because we are talking about benefit, we imply that the aided result of our laboratory testing is being compared with some unaided results. These unaided results are sometimes gathered before the fitting of hearing aids, and sometimes they are gathered on the same appointment that the aided testing is conducted. The primary purpose of laboratory measures of outcome is to demonstrate that hearing aids are providing a reasonable amount of benefit, provide reassurance to the patient that certain features on the hearing aids are operating adequately, or to troubleshoot patient complaints. Lab measures of outcome are completed in the aided condition and compared with those of the unaided condition. Since many of the tests listed below do not have published norms, you would have to collect data on a group of subjects of similar ages to your patients with normal or near-normal hearing. These norms would serve as a point of comparison with those of the patients in whom you are conducting the lab measures.

Since most lab measures can be expressed in a percent correct score, the results are easy to gather and discuss with patients. The chief limitation of lab measures of outcome is that they are gathered in a contrived listening environment (usually your sound booth) and the results are often not reflective of real-world listening experiences; therefore, you need to be cautious about how you interpret the results of lab measures. They can offer reassurance and guidance on the quality of the fitting, but good results in your test booth do not equate to a successful fitting in the real world. Here are some examples of laboratory measures of outcome to consider using in your clinic as a way to cross-check self-reports of outcome, which are discussed in the next section of this chapter.

- Count-the-Dots Aided Audiogram (Functional Gain)
- Aided Word or Sentence Recognition in Quiet
- Aided Word or Sentence Recognition in Noise

- Aided Audibility (QuickSIN presented at 50 dB HL in the sound field)
- Aided Acceptable Noise Test
- Sound Quality Judgments.

SELF-REPORTS OF HEARING AID OUTCOME

Self-reports (questionnaires) of hearing aid outcome have been developed and utilized over the past few decades. Patients have always provided clinicians with real-world assessments of outcomes from their hearing aids, and frequently these reports were used for counseling and hearing aid adjustments. Until recently, however, most real-world assessments of outcome involved informal discussions between the patient and the professional. Rather than formally measuring real-world outcomes, professionals relied more heavily on laboratory measures of fitting outcomes. These measures included speech recognition in quiet and in noise, functional or insertion gain measures, and aided loudness judgments. In the past 20 years, however, several well-designed and validated self-assessment inventories have been introduced. The goal now is to make these inventories part of the routine hearing aid fitting protocol. Self-report outcome measures with known psychometric properties are useful for determining the effectiveness of hearing aids. Effectiveness with amplification can be measured across several dimensions, including handicap reduction, acceptance, benefit, and satisfaction. Several self-report measures of hearing aid outcome have been developed over the past two decades addressing each of these dimensions. Because they comprise two of the most significant components of a patient's experience with hearing aids, only self-report measures of hearing aid benefit and satisfaction are discussed.

An important question to address at this time is, "Why do we need self-report measures of real-world outcome?" There are at least three reasons that are related to quality. First, for largely economic reasons, health care is becoming more consumer driven. In this evolving system, the consumer decides what treatment is selected and when it is complete. The major index of quality of service is self-report outcome and satisfaction. Consumer-driven health care places an added emphasis on the patient's point of view; therefore, it is critical to measure the real-world benefit and satisfaction of hearing aid use. Because today's patients are, on average, more savvy and better informed than their grandparents, they want to know how much benefit they are receiving in everyday listening situations. Using a self-report of hearing aid outcome allows you to measure and report to the patient how they are doing compared with an average.

A second reason self-report measures of outcome are gaining importance is related to the fact that many of these real-world experiences simply cannot be measured effectively in laboratory conditions. The traditional hearing aid outcome measures clinicians have used in the past, such as speech recognition in quiet and in noise, do not capture the true experiences of hearing aid use in everyday listening situations. Consider hearing aids with automatic and adaptive directional technology. The effectiveness of features such as this depend heavily on the lifestyle and listening conditions of the individual patient. In order to quantify the true impact that hearing loss and its associated treatment have on activity limitations, lifestyles, and so forth, self-report outcome measures can be used.

Third, even when laboratory conditions are used to simulate real-world listening situations, they do not always resemble the patient's impression of the actual real-life situation. Self-report outcome measures are increasing in use because they give us a scientifically defensible way to validly measure the real-life success of the hearing aid fitting.

Finally, evidence-based practice has become a standard component in the clinical decision-making process. An evidence-based-practice paradigm requires that clinicians demonstrate that their hearing aid fittings are providing benefit in real-world conditions. For this reason, self-reports of outcome are the new gold standard for measuring and reporting success. Self-report measures of hearing aid benefit and satisfaction are reviewed below.

There are two major types of self-reports or questionnaires that can be administered. One type is called open ended and the other is called closed ended.

@CONNECT

Why Self-Report Outcome Measures Need to Be Part of Your Best Practice

1. Comparison of different dispensing sites or personnel: You are the manager of a hearing aid dispensing practice that has two offices. You fit the same hearing aids in both offices. Are the patients in Office A as satisfied with their hearing aids as the patients fitted at Office B?
2. Comparison of different fitting procedures: You always fit your hearing aids to the NAL-NL2 targets with careful verification and adjustment using probe-microphone measures. Your partner simply uses the manufacturer's first-fit setting. Will both groups of patients have the same benefit and satisfaction with hearing aids in the real world? A recent report by Abrams and colleagues (2012) suggests that the two approaches lead to different outcomes!
3. Comparison of circuitry: Your favorite manufacturers just added a new noise-reduction feature, which adds several hundred dollars to the cost of the hearing aids. If your patients were fitted with that feature, would they observe improved speech understanding in noise in their everyday-use situations?
4. Counseling effectiveness: You have decided to conduct a free morning counseling session each Saturday for all of your patients who have a high ANL test score and poor QuickSIN performance (e.g., patients considered "at risk"). Will this extra effort result in improved real-world satisfaction and benefit with their hearing aids?
5. Documentation of service effectiveness: You know you do a good job, but do you have data to prove it? Are your patients more satisfied than the average person fitted with hearing aids? How often do their IOI-HA scores exceed national norms? How often are their COSI goals obtained?

6. Research has shown that patients are significantly more satisfied with their hearing aids when they have been given a formalized outcome measure asking them if they are satisfied with their hearing aids.

Open-Ended Self-Report Measures of Outcome

Open-ended self-report measures are those that allow the patient to nominate and target their own areas of expected improvement with amplification. The assumed advantage of an open-ended scale is that it can be tailored to the true communication needs of the individual patient. In other words, if you and the patient work together carefully, the items selected will represent truly difficult listening situations for that patient, rather than arbitrary listening situations collected from "average" patients. The downside of these open-ended questionnaires is that it makes it difficult to compare your patient's performance to a large pool of other hearing aid users, as the specific listening situations they nominated might be unique.

Client Oriented Scale of Improvement

The Client Oriented Scale of Improvement (COSI) (Figure 3–7) was developed by the National Acoustic Laboratories in 1997. The COSI is an open-ended scale in which the patient targets up to five listening situations for improvement with amplification (e.g., listening to television when there is background noise, talking on the phone with my grandchildren, etc.). The COSI was normalized on 1,770 adults with hearing loss is Australia. The goal of the COSI is for the patient to target specific listening situations when the hearing aids are fitted, and to report the degree of benefit obtained after a few weeks of hearing aid use. It is important to have patients nominate situations that are common and long-standing, as many times they will want to focus on

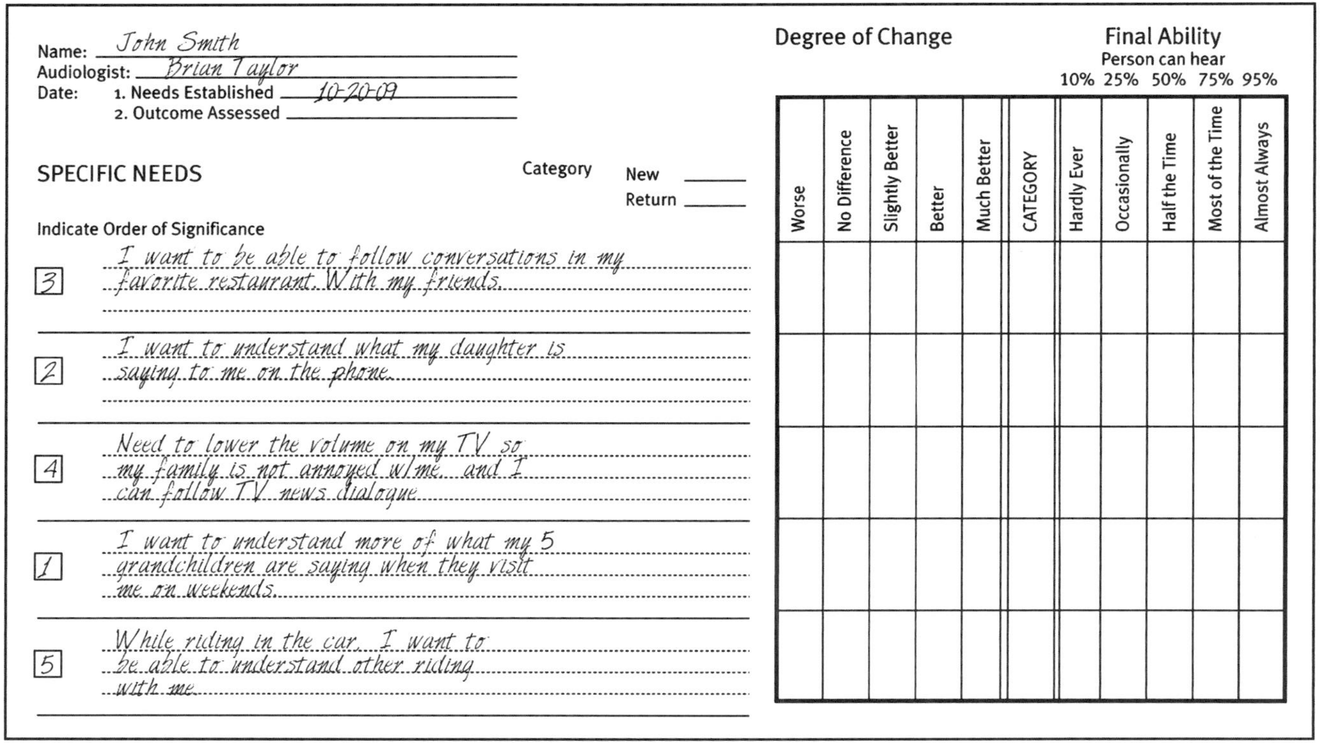

Name: _John Smith_

Audiologist: _Brian Taylor_ 1. Needs Established _10-20-09_

Date: _____ 2. Outcome Assessed _____

Category New _____
          Return _____

SPECIFIC NEEDS

Indicate Order of Significance

Degree of Change							Final Ability Person can hear
	Worse	No Difference	Slightly Better	Better	Much Better	CATEGORY	Hardly Ever / Occasionally / Half the Time / Most of the Time / Almost Always

Final Ability Person can hear: 10% 25% 50% 75% 95%
Hardly Ever · Occasionally · Half the Time · Most of the Time · Almost Always

[3] I want to be able to follow conversations in my favorite restaurant with my friends.

[2] I want to understand what my daughter is saying to me on the phone.

[4] Need to lower the volume on my TV so my family is not annoyed w/ me, and I can follow TV news dialogue.

[1] I want to understand more of what my 5 grandchildren are saying when they visit me on weekends.

[5] While riding in the car, I want to be able to understand other riding with me.

Figure 3–7. Client Oriented Scale of Improvement (COSI), which was developed by the National Acoustic Laboratories in Australia in the 1990s.

"current events." The first two items (in importance) will probably give you the best "read" regarding the success of the fitting. The findings then can be generally compared with those expected for the population in similar listening situations. The findings can be scored as "Degree of Change," "Final Ability," or both.

Many hearing aid manufacturers now include the COSI in their fitting software. The COSI can also be downloaded from the NAL at http://www.nal.gov.au/. The COSI has become one of the most commonly used real-world measures of benefit among dispensers. This is partly because of the "personalization" that we have discussed, but also because it is very easy to administer and score, and is quite "low tech" (in desperation, you could get by with a pencil and bar napkin!).

Glasgow Hearing Aid Benefit Profile

The Glasgow Hearing Aid Benefit Profile (GHABP) examines six dimensions of hearing aid outcome: disability, handicap, hearing aid use, benefit, satisfaction, and residual disability. The GHABP consists of four predetermined and four patient-nominated items; therefore, the GHABP could be considered a combination open-ended and closed-ended measure of outcome. This is an advantage for patients who have trouble thinking of specific situations on their own. The GHABP was normalized on 293 adults. Based on the normative findings, it is an appropriate instrument for clinicians who want to use self-report data to measure improvement in audibility. The Hearing Aid Benefit Interview, a completely open-ended questionnaire, is the precursor to the GHABP (Gatehouse, 1994). The GHABP can be downloaded at http://www.ihr.mrc.ac.uk/.

Closed-Ended Self-Report Measures of Outcome

Closed-ended self-report measures allow the patient to complete a self-report scale using a predetermined list of areas of concern. The primary advantage of the closed-ended scale is that the scores can be more readily compared with normative data. In other words, your patient in Cairo, Illinois, or Paris, Texas, is answering the very same questions as a new hearing aid user in New York City. This provides a large database, allowing for comparisons with considerable hearing aid data and demographic data. One of the disadvantages of a closed-ended measure is that individual communication preferences cannot be accounted for. In an era in which outcome measures are gaining importance, this is an important consideration. Closed-ended outcome measures, although outstanding tools for conducting clinical research, are sometimes difficult to use to address the unique needs of all individuals seen in the clinic. The next sections provide an overview of some of the most popular closed-ended surveys.

Abbreviated Profile of Hearing Aid Benefit

In an attempt to develop a more clinic-friendly measure of outcome, the Abbreviated Profile of Hearing Aid Benefit (APHAB) was developed (Table 3–1). Like the COSI, which we discussed previously, it is a measure of benefit rather than satisfaction. The goal of the APHAB is to quantify the disability caused by hearing loss, and the reduction of that disability achieved with hearing aids. The APHAB uses 24 items covering four subscales: ease of communication (listening in quiet), reverberation, background noise, and aversiveness to sounds. It can be used to measure unaided or aided "percent of problems" or hearing aid benefit (the difference between unaided and aided). The APHAB has been normalized on 128 adults with mild to moderate hearing loss.

The APHAB is the most commonly used outcome measure in hearing aid research. It is probably the most commonly used closed-set outcome measure used among dispensers, too, although the overall-use rate is disappointingly low. While the administration and scoring is relatively simple, it is more detailed than some of the other scales. Several hearing aid manufacturers have the APHAB and the automated scoring as part of their fitting software. The APHAB can be downloaded at http://www.ausp.memphis.edu/harl/aphab.html/.

Table 3–1. Published Norms for the Abbreviated Profile of Hearing Aid Benefit (*APHAB*) for Wide Dynamic Range Compression (WDRC)-Capable Hearing Aids

Users of WDRC-Capable Hearing Aids—Unaided				
Percentile	EC	RV	BN	AV
95	99	99	99	70
80	83	87	89	35
65	75	81	81	21
50	63	71	75	14
35	56	65	67	9
20	46	58	58	3
5	26	47	41	1
Users of WDRC-Capable Hearing Aids—Aided				
Percentile	EC	RV	BN	AV
95	86	79	82	82
80	39	57	58	64
65	29	46	49	53
50	23	37	40	38
35	17	29	32	23
20	12	21	22	14
5	5	12	14	2
Users of WDRC-Capable Hearing Aids—Benefit				
Percentile	EC	RV	BN	AV
95	76	70	56	16
80	52	52	47	0
65	46	41	39	−8
50	38	34	33	−13
35	29	27	23	−25
20	19	16	12	−41
5	−10	−3	−1	−61

Note: The *APHAB* was developed at the University of Memphis.

@CONNECT

Benchmarking: Self-Report Norms and Critical Differences

Choosing an outcome measure that has published norms and critical difference values is important to the clinical management process. The norms tell you how your patient compares with other patients of similar demographics. The critical difference values allow the clinician to make a statement of true difference in scores, as with the speech perception testing discussed previously in this chapter. For an example of this, we use the Abbreviated Profile of Hearing Aid Benefit (APHAB) as it is one of the most popular self-assessment inventories. It provides for both pretest and posttest administration. The APHAB has four subscales: Easy Communication (EC) listening environments, Background Noise (BN) listening environments, Reverberation (RV) listening environments, and Aversive (AV) listening experiences. Scores are calculated for each subscale (a computer program available with the inventory makes the scoring and interpretation very straightforward). The prefitting and postfitting items are identical; the patient is simply instructed to respond (initially) as though they were not using amplification. Alternatively, some clinicians use the pretest administration to determine the status with current or old hearing aids to compare with newly acquired hearing aids. In any event, the patient is asked to respond to the 24 items by answering what percent of the time they experience the scenario of the items. Examples of items include:

- Traffic noises are too loud . . .
- When I am talking with someone across a large empty room, I understand the words . . .
- When I am in a small office, interviewing or answering questions, I have difficulty following the conversation . . .

A Always (99 to 100% of the time)
B Almost Always (87% of the time)
C Generally (75% of the time)
D Half the time (50% of the time)
E Occasionally (25% of the time)
F Seldom (12% of the time)
G Never (0 to 1% of the time)

Upon completion of the inventory, the prefitting scores might look like this: EC: 65, RV: 80, BN: 90, AV: 15. By looking at the table of norms, it can be readily discerned that the patient is at approximately the 50th percentile for EC, RV, and AV subscales, but closer to the 90th percentile for the BN subscale. Translated into language that would be useful in counseling and management planning: The patient performs similarly to others with her hearing loss in three of the subscales (EC, RV, and AV) but has considerably more trouble with background noise than her comparison group, that is, her responses indicate that she has trouble in background noise about 90% of the time. According to the normative table, that would place her at the 80th percentile, that is, 80% of her peers have less trouble in background noise. Stated another way, only 20% of her peers have *more* trouble in background noise. Now, following the issuance of hearing aids and several weeks of adjustment to the hearing aids, you repeat the APHAB (the aided version). For this administration you obtain scores of EC: 15, RV: 30, BN: 30, and AV: 50. Again, referring to the table of norms Aided Condition, these scores indicate that the patient is at approximately the 35th percentile for EC, RV, and BN, and the 50th percentile for AV. Translated into language that would be useful in counseling and management planning: The patient has fewer problems in the listening situations (EC, RV, and BN) than 65% of her peers (100 minus 35 equals 65) but has about the same amount of trouble with aversive sounds as about 50% of her peers (i.e., scores at the 50th percentile). The difference between the unaided and aided scores derives the benefit score, that is, EC: 50, RV: 50, BN: 60, and AV: −35. One more time, looking at the table of norms for *benefit* it is obvious that our patient's benefit scores put her at approximately the 80th percentile for EC and RV. Interpolating the percentile for the BN subscale suggests that she is actually up at the 90th percentile for benefit obtained in noisy environments. Pat yourself on the back for doing a "good job." But wait! The AV subscale puts her at approximately the 25th percentile for benefit with aversive sounds. That subscale can be a bit tricky to interpret. Most hearing aid users tend to have a "worse score" (negative benefit) when the aided scores are compared with the unaided scores. This score might simply imply that she is now hearing some of those louder sounds as loud sounds (they should be!), compared with the unaided condition where they might have been less annoying. On the other hand, it might indicate that the MPO is set too high for real-life aversive sounds.

Profile of Aided Loudness

Up to this point, we have discussed outcome measures that primarily have been designed to measure hearing aid benefit—that is, do the hearing aids help the patient communicate in the real world? A related, but different, aspect of the hearing aid fitting is providing the appropriate gain for soft, average, and loud inputs—making soft sounds soft, average sounds comfortable, and loud sounds loud, but not too loud. Recall that we talked about this in our discussion of wide dynamic range compression (WDRC), and matching probe-microphone targets. It is reasonable, therefore, to also conduct a real-world subjective measure to determine if indeed aided loudness perceptions are appropriate. That is the purpose of the Profile of Aided Loudness (PAL) (Figure 3–8).

The PAL consists of 12 items, all relatively common environmental sounds, four each in the soft, average, and loud categories. The patient scores the loudness rating for each of these

7. The dryer running

Loudness rating	Satisfaction rating
0 Do not hear	5. Just right
1 Very soft	4. Pretty good
2 Soft	3. Okay
3 Comfortable, but slightly soft	2. Not too good
4 Comfortable	1. Not good at all
5 Comfortable, but slightly loud	
6 Loud, but OK	
7 Uncomfortably loud	

8. You chewing soft food

Loudness rating	Satisfaction rating
0 Do not hear	5. Just right
1 Very soft	4. Pretty good
2 Soft	3. Okay
3 Comfortable, but slightly soft	2. Not too good
4 Comfortable	1. Not good at all
5 Comfortable, but slightly loud	
6 Loud, but OK	
7 Uncomfortably loud	

9. Listening to a marching band

Loudness rating	Satisfaction rating
0 Do not hear	5. Just right
1 Very soft	4. Pretty good
2 Soft	3. Okay
3 Comfortable, but slightly soft	2. Not too good
4 Comfortable	1. Not good at all
5 Comfortable, but slightly loud	
6 Loud, but OK	
7 Uncomfortably loud	

10. A barking dog

Loudness rating	Satisfaction rating
0 Do not hear	5. Just right
1 Very soft	4. Pretty good
2 Soft	3. Okay
3 Comfortable, but slightly soft	2. Not too good
4 Comfortable	1. Not good at all
5 Comfortable, but slightly loud	
6 Loud, but OK	
7 Uncomfortably loud	

11. A lawn mower

Loudness rating	Satisfaction rating
0 Do not hear	5. Just right
1 Very soft	4. Pretty good
2 Soft	3. Okay
3 Comfortable, but slightly soft	2. Not too good
4 Comfortable	1. Not good at all
5 Comfortable, but slightly loud	
6 Loud, but OK	
7 Uncomfortably loud	

12. A microwave buzzer sounding

Loudness rating	Satisfaction rating
0 Do not hear	5. Just right
1 Very soft	4. Pretty good
2 Soft	3. Okay
3 Comfortable, but slightly soft	2. Not too good
4 Comfortable	1. Not good at all
5 Comfortable, but slightly loud	
6 Loud, but OK	
7 Uncomfortably loud	

Take an average score for soft, average, and loud sounds and compare the scores to the average scores of normally hearing individuals. The patient summary sheet is used for this type of scoring. In this manner, the clinician may compare unaided loudness perception to aided loudness perception as well as having a numeric target for the aided condition.

PATIENT SUMMARY
Profile of Aided Loudness (PAL)
Unaided Performance

Soft sounds	Q3	Q4	Q5	Q8	Category average
Loudness	___	___	___	___	___ (target = 2)
Satisfaction	___	___	___	___	
Average sounds	Q1	Q6	Q7	Q12	Category average
Loudness	___	___	___	___	___ (target = 4)
Satisfaction	___	___	___	___	
Loud sounds	Q2	Q9	Q10	Q11	Category average
Loudness	___	___	___	___	___ (target = 6)
Satisfaction	___	___	___	___	

Aided Performance

Soft sounds	Q3	Q4	Q5	Q8	Category average
Loudness	___	___	___	___	___ (target = 2)
Satisfaction	___	___	___	___	
Average sounds	Q1	Q6	Q7	Q12	Category average
Loudness	___	___	___	___	___ (target = 4)
Satisfaction	___	___	___	___	
Loud sounds	Q2	Q9	Q10	Q11	Category average
Loudness	___	___	___	___	___ (target = 6)
Satisfaction	___	___	___	___	

Figure 3–8. Profile of Aided Loudness (PAL) is shown.

sounds (usually aided, but could be conducted both unaided and aided) using the seven-point loudness anchors of the Cox Contour Test. The patient also rates their satisfaction for the loudness on a five-point scale (1 = very satisfied). For example, your patient might rate the "beep" of a microwave #4 for loudness, but only #3 for satisfaction. The loudness rating of #4 is great (just like patient with normal hearing), but why is the patient not satisfied? It is probably because for the past 20 years the loudness perception of the beep was only a #2, and now at #4 it is annoying. This clearly is now a counseling issue, not a "turn down the gain" issue. But how would you have known without the PAL findings? If a patient simply said "My microwave is too loud" some dispensers would be tempted to make hearing aid adjustments.

The PAL is easy to administer and score, and provides information not available from other self-assessment scales (although the AV scale of the APHAB should agree with the four loud items of the PAL).

Hearing Handicap Inventory for Adults and Hearing Handicap Inventory for the Elderly

So far we have mostly discussed measuring the benefit of hearing aids—reduction of disability—but we also are concerned with the reduction of handicap. Although the two usually go hand in hand, it certainly is possible to have a handicap without a disability. There are two scales that commonly have been used to measure hearing handicap, and the resulting effects of hearing aid treatment. The original scale was the Hearing Handicap Inventory for the Elderly (HHIE) (elderly meaning people over the age of 65 years) which was then modified for younger adults and called the Hearing Handicap Inventory for Adults (HHIA) (administered to people under the age of 65 years). The HHIE/ HHIA were designed to both quantify handicap and also assess benefit by measuring change in perceived handicap after the fitting of hearing aids. Both scales have a 25-item version and a 10-item screening version. They also both have two subscales: emotional consequences and social and situational effects. The goal of these scales is to measure the perceived effects of hearing loss. Both the HHIE and the HHIA allow the patient to answer "yes," "no," or "sometimes" to all 25 items on the questionnaire. The higher the total score, the greater the hearing handicap. The scale is designed so that even people with normal hearing may answer "2" for some items (e.g., Do you have difficulty hearing when someone speaks in a whisper?"). Some dispensers have used this tool in the unaided format to gain insight as to whether a patient is a candidate for amplification. If a person has a 30 to 50 dB hearing loss, but their self-reported HHIE score is only 8, one might question whether they need (or are ready to accept) hearing aids.

Satisfaction with Amplification in Daily Life

Up to this point, we have mostly discussed tests of hearing aid benefit, but as mentioned previously, it is also important to assess satisfaction with hearing aids. The Satisfaction with Amplification in Daily Life (SADL) was designed to quantify satisfaction with hearing aids using 15 items in four subscales. It is a companion test to an expectations questionnaire titled the ECHO (Expected Consequences of Hearing Aid Ownership). The four subscales of the SADL consist of positive effects, service and costs, negative features, and personal image. Each item is rated on a five-point scale ranging from A = not at all; B = a little; F = greatly; to G = tremendously. The SADL was normalized on between 126 and 225 adults depending on the subscale, and can be downloaded at http://www.ausp.memphis.edu/harl/sadl.html/.

Device Oriented Subjective Outcome Scale

Research indicates that final hearing aid outcome is influenced by the personality or social style of the patient. For example, patients who display personality traits in which they have a willingness to please others are more likely to report higher outcomes relative to other personality types. For this reason the Device Oriented Subjective Outcome Scale (DOSO) questionnaire was developed to measure hearing aid outcomes in a manner that is relatively independent of wearer personality. Patients choose from several responses to indicate how well the hearing aids work to accomplish specific goals. The DOSO produces scores for six subscales: Speech Cues, Listening Effort, Pleasantness, Quietness, Convenience, and Use. The DOSO is available for download at http://www.memphis.edu/csd/harl/doso.htm/.

Hearing Aid Performance Inventory

The Hearing Aid Performance Inventory (HAPI) (Walden, Demorest, & Helper, 1984) uses 64 items based on 12 bipolar communication features (e.g., visual cues present/absent). The goal of the HAPI is to assess the effectiveness of amplification on a variety of everyday listening situations. The HAPI has been normalized on 128 hearing aid users, 119 of whom were men.

Speech, Spatial and Qualities of Hearing Scale

The Speech, Spatial and Qualities of Hearing Scale (SSQ) is designed to measure a range of hearing disabilities across several domains, including auditory disability and handicap. There are 80 questions about auditory attention, perceptions of distance and movement, sound-source segregation, listening effort, prosody, and sound quality. The SSQ is designed to be administered to patients through an interview format (similar to the COSI or GHABP), rather than self-administered. The SSQ has gained popularity recently, especially in Europe. Recently, a shorter version of the SSQ has been introduced to the market. It can downloaded at http://www.ihr.gla.ac.uk/products/ssq.php/.

International Outcome Inventory—Hearing Aid (IOI-HA)

To this point, we have discussed various scales that have been designed primarily to assess a specific aspect of hearing aid outcome: benefit, reduction of handicap, loudness normalization, satisfaction, and so forth. It is cumbersome and time-consuming to conduct five or six different inventories, and some have suggested that a single "screening" inventory could be used to cover many areas in a single form. Maybe one does not have to ask 10 or more questions about benefit to determine if someone is indeed obtaining benefit? Consisting of seven questions on a five-point rating scale, the goal of the International Outcome Inventory–Hearing Aid (IOI-HA) (Figure 3–9), therefore, is to assess benefit, satisfaction, and quality-of-life changes associated with hearing aid use. The creators of the IOI-HA determined that the seven questions could be grouped into two separate factors. Factor 1, which is questions 1, 2, 4, and 7, is interpreted

International Outcome Inventory for Hearing Aids (IOI-HA)

1. Think about how much you used your present hearing aid(s) over the past two weeks. On an average day, how many hours did you use the hearing aid(s)?

none	less than 1 hour a day	1 to 4 hours a day	4 to 8 hours a day	more than 8 hours a day
☐	☐	☐	☐	☐

2. Think about the situation where you most wanted to hear better, before you got your present hearing aid(s). Over the past two weeks, how much has the hearing aid helped in those situations?

helped not at all	helped slightly	helped moderately	helped quite a lot	helped very much
☐	☐	☐	☐	☐

3. Think again about the situation where you most wanted to hear better. When you use your present hearing aid(s), how much difficulty do you STILL have in that situation?

very much difficulty	quite a lot of difficulty	moderate difficulty	Slight difficulty	no difficulty
☐	☐	☐	☐	☐

4. Considering everything, do you think your present hearing aid(s) is worth the trouble?

not at all worth it	Slightly worth it	Moderately worth it	quite a lot worth it	very much worth it
☐	☐	☐	☐	☐

5. Over the past two weeks, with your present hearing aid(s), how much have your hearing difficulties affected the things you can do?

affected very much	affected quite a lot	affected moderately	affected slightly	affected not at all
☐	☐	☐	☐	☐

6. Over the past two weeks, with your present hearing aid(s), how much do you think other people were bothered by your hearing difficulties?

bothered very much	bothered quite a lot	bothered moderately	bothered slightly	bothered not at all
☐	☐	☐	☐	☐

7. Considering everything, how much has your present hearing aid(s) changed your enjoyment of life?

worse	no change	slightly better	quite a lot better	Very much better
☐	☐	☐	☐	☐

8. How much hearing difficulty do you have when you are **not** wearing a hearing aid?

severe	moderately-severe	moderate	mild	none
☐	☐	☐	☐	☐

Figure 3–9. International Outcome Inventory—Hearing Aid (IOI-HA) is shown.

as encompassing introspection about the hearing aids ("me and my hearing aids"). Factor 2, comprising questions 3, 5, and 6, is interpreted as reflecting the influence of the hearing aids on the individual's interactions with the outside world ("me and the rest of the world").

The IOI-HA was designed primarily to be used as a supplement to other self-report tools and, because at the outset it was made available in over 20 languages, it also would serve as a way to compare hearing aid outcomes around the world using the same self-assessment tool. Many dispensers, however, use it as a stand-alone measure of the quality of the fitting, since it does cover many important aspects. It can be downloaded (all languages) at http://www.ausp.memphis.edu/harl/ioiha.html/.

Since hearing aid outcome takes on several dimensions, you need to measure it with more than one questionnaire or test. When you consider that the World Health Organization's definition of outcome comprises at least four domains, combined with the fact that there are laboratory and real-world components to outcome, it becomes a little overwhelming to determine which outcome measure may give clinicians the best "bang for the buck." Humes (2012) summarized three separate domains of outcome. His work gives us the best path toward comprehensive assessment of hearing aid outcome that is feasible to implement in the clinic. According to Humes the three domains of hearing aid outcome are benefaction (a combination of benefit and satisfaction), usage, and aided speech recognition. These domains are represented in Figure 3–10 with the relative weighting of each on final outcome of the hearing aid fitting corresponding to the size of the oval in the figure. Clinicians would be wise to incorporate the findings of Humes into clinical practice by routinely conducting a measure of benefaction, usage, and aided speech recognition into their assessment of outcome. Some specific tools with respect to measuring these three domains of outcome are also represented in Figure 3–10.

SEMISTRUCTURED INTERVIEWS AND JOURNALING

A complementary approach to the administration of an established self-report measure like those mentioned previously is the use of a semistructured interview and journaling. Although

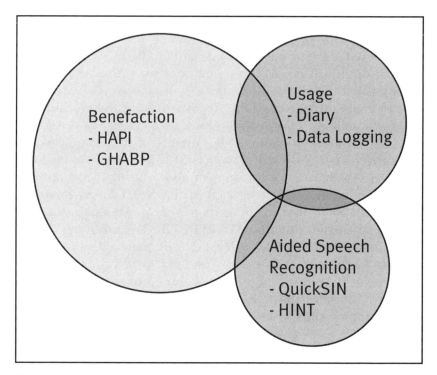

Figure 3–10. Humes circles are shown. *HAPI*, Hearing Aid Performance Inventory; *GHABP*, Glasgow Hearing Aid Benefit Profile; *Quick-SIN*, Quick Speech-in-Noise test; *HINT*, Hearing-in-Noise Test.

there is a paucity of clinical studies underscoring the effectiveness of semistructured interviews or journaling as methods of documenting outcome, both serve as reasonable compliments to traditional self-report measures of hearing aid outcome.

A semistructured interview format warrants the use of closed-set questions. Typically, these closed-set questions would be asked at the hearing aid follow-up appointment (1 to 4 weeks post fitting) and they allow the audiologist to quantify the patient's attitude toward hearing aid use. An example of a semistructured interview question would be "Thinking about your hearing aid use of the last two to four weeks (since you were fitted with them), have you or your family noticed a difference in your communication ability?" Using a closed-set format, the patient would be asked to respond "yes," "no," or "unsure." Devising a series of similar closed-set questions, allows the audiologist to quantify patient attitude toward hearing aid use and generates additional patient dialogue.

Journaling is another method in which audiologists can quantify hearing aid fitting outcomes. At the end of the initial hearing aid fitting appointment, the patient is given a journal (or diary) that the patient is encouraged to use on a daily basis in order to document their feelings and outlook toward amplification. When constructing a patient journal you need to provide the patient with enough space to record at least 14 days' worth of entries. Each day the patient would be expected to set aside a few minutes to complete a journal entry. The following questions can be used effectively in a patient journal and can be reviewed with the audiologist at the subsequent follow-up appointment:

- How many hours did you wear your instruments today?
- Describe the situations where the instruments were effective.
- Describe the situations where the instruments fell short of your expectations.
- On a 1 to 10 scale (ten being the best) how would you rate your ability to communicate TODAY with your instruments?
- What other comments come to mind about your hearing aid use today?

OUTCOME AND QUALITY

From the perspective of quality, outcome measures are used to improve delivery of services. Here is a simple method for gaining an understanding of how outcomes and best practices are intertwined:

1. Implement a comprehensive clinical protocol like the ones described in this chapter.
2. Choose two or three different self-reports that measure "benefaction" in a comprehensive manner. One of the outcome measures ought to measure overall patient satisfaction of the clinical experience. A patient comment card does this.

Another outcome measure needs to be real-world benefit. The APHAB and COSI are two examples of benefit measures. Lastly, other facets of outcome not directly measured with a comment card or benefit scale, such as reduction in handicap and quality of life, can be measured with another questionnaire. The IOI-HA is an excellent tool to measure some of these other dimensions of outcome.

3. Establish benchmarks by using either published normative data (e.g., on the APHAB, scoring in the 80th percentile on the four aided subscales is a reasonable benchmark) or create your own benchmarks by collecting data on at least 30 patients. (Six Sigma experts suggest that you are very likely to obtain a representative sample of your population when you have collected data from 30 or more individuals.)

4. Set up a computerized office management system (e.g., Aud-Serv office management system) so that patients can directly enter the self-report data into the office management system. Computerizing your outcome measures saves a lot of time collecting data and makes the data analysis very easy.

5. Once you have established benchmarks (norms) you can begin to compare the results collected from the patients with your measures of outcome. Using a computerized office management system, you can enter outcome data and compare it with your benchmarks.

6. Once a month compare the outcome data in the aggregate to the normative benchmark data. Look for gaps in the data you have collected as compared with the benchmarks.

7. A gap is a red flag that a process improvement might be needed (e.g., if your data from dozens of patients are showing a lower score on the background noise [BN] subscale of the APHAB, this suggests that you need to perform a root-cause analysis of possible reasons for this gap).

8. Conduct a root-cause analysis by brainstorming all the possible reasons for a gap in the BN subscale. This list could include product defects, insufficient counseling of patient, lack of objective verification measures on directional microphones measures, and several others. Identify one or two strong possibilities for the gap and create a plan of action for improvement. This will likely include the need to update a

clinical process (e.g., add more counseling time or complete additional testing of the patient) or perhaps more training of the staff.

9. Continue to collect and analyze outcome data and compare them with your benchmarked data on a monthly basis. Quality is a never ending cyclical process.

PRACTICAL ISSUES RELATED TO THE USE OF SELF-REPORT MEASURES

In order to make this review of outcome measures more useful for the busy clinician, several commonly asked questions are posed, along with recommendations.

When Should a Self-Report of Outcome Be Given to the Patient?

The question of exactly when a self-report of outcome should be administered to a patient is important for two reasons. One, if the self-report is completed too soon, the patient may not have had enough time to become familiar with the fundamental daily care and maintenance of the devices, such as cleaning and insertion/removal into the ears. At least one study asserts that administering self-reports too soon results in artificially lower-than-expected outcomes because patients were not given ample time to learn how to use their hearing aids.

On the other hand, if a clinician waits too long to conduct self-report measures, the entire fitting process is unnecessarily prolonged. Both the patient and the clinician are needlessly waiting to bring closure to the fitting process. A recent evidence-based review of hearing aid acclimatization suggests that hearing aid benefit is optimized approximately 30 days post-fitting for the typical patient. The clinical evidence suggests that self-reports of outcome should be administered about 3 to 4 weeks post-fitting.

What Self-Report Outcome Measure Should Be Used?

Due to the abundance of self-reports available to the clinician, it is difficult to know which ones work best. When making this decision, it is important to examine exactly what dimension of real-world outcome you are trying to capture in the most time-efficient manner. Cox and Alexander (2007), in a large-scale study with several variables, examined the relationship between self-reports of outcome and personality. Analyses of the collection of outcome measures produced a set of three components that were interpreted as a Device component, a Success component, and an Acceptance component. Results suggest that personality is more closely linked to self-report of hearing aid outcome than conventional laboratory measures, such as the audiogram. Precisely how personality affects outcome should be taken into consideration when selecting a self-report questionnaire.

How Does Validation and Verification Affect Quality?

Before answering this question, let us make sure we are on the same page with respect to the terms "validation" and "verification." In simple terms verification is ensuring that you are meeting a documented standard (matching a prescriptive target using probe-microphone measures), while validation is ensuring that the patient is benefiting (and is satisfied) with the settings you have prescribed. After reading this chapter, you should have a good understanding of how each procedure contributes to the final result. Kochkin (2011) reported that the routine use of both standardized verification and validation procedures, such as the ones outlined in this chapter, results in fewer patient visits. Considering that fewer patient visits results in better clinical efficiency and that better clinical efficiency is a foundation of quality, these data suggest that validation and verification contribute to improved quality. According to Kochkin just 35% of patients report having received both validation and verification of their fitting. Furthermore, patients receiving both procedures had a mean total of 2.41 patient visits for a fitting, while patients receiving neither verification nor validation had a mean total of 3.57 patient visits for their fitting. These results certainly indicate that both verification and validation need to be completed early in the patient journey.

THE FOLLOW-UP APPOINTMENT

In many ways the follow-up appointment, which is stage 6 of the patient journey, is the forgotten component of the clinical experience. Since many patients have adequately adjusted to amplification by the time periodic follow-up appointments are scheduled, this appointment is often anticlimactic. The typical follow-up appointment is about 20 to 30 minutes in duration and usually involves routine cleaning and checking of the hearing instruments, some counseling and maybe some tweaking or troubleshooting of the devices using fitting software.

Recent research has shown that periodic "face time" with the patient is likely to result in both an improved outlook toward communication and better hearing aid utilization following informational counseling sessions. Saunders and Forsline (2012) evaluated two different types of counseling sessions and their impact on outcomes for two groups of experienced hearing aids users. One group was provided information counseling, which was a general explanation of test results, encouragement to discuss experiences relative to communication with hearing aids and recommendation about how to more effectively use their devices. The second group was provided performance-perceptual counseling (PPC). PPC requires the audiologist to measure speech recognition in noise ability objectively and then subjectively. Patients that overestimate their ability to understand speech in the presence of noise are counseled differently than those that underestimate their ability to understand speech in the presence of noise. The authors also used several standardized self-reports of outcome as well as a semistructured interview to measure the results of these two different types of counseling. Responses to the semistructured interview questions showed both types of counseling had a beneficial effect on patient's outlook toward communication and benefit from amplification. These findings suggest that periodic follow-up appointments that provide information on communication repair strategies and dialogue on how to cope with hearing loss and hearing aid use serve to enhance the benefit and quality of life that result from amplification—even for patients with hearing instruments older than five years.

Customizing the Follow-Up

Another important component of the follow-up appointment process is the patient's use of auditory training. Auditory training is best described as a series of regimented exercises designed to take advantage of the neuroplasticity of the brain. As previously mentioned, Saunders (2012) evaluated the effectiveness of Listening and Communication Enhancement Exercises (LACE), which is one commercially available type of auditory training and found that regimented auditory training exercises did not improve patient outcomes for the most patient. One take away from this research is that clinicians are encouraged to collaborate with patients to identify the type of follow-up program that will optimize patient outcomes and utilization. In addition to information counseling that addresses communication strategies and orientation to hearing aid use, clinicians can offer Performance-Perceptual Counseling or aural rehabilitation classes. Customizing the specific type of follow-up service can be accomplished using a shared-decision making approach, like the one outlined earlier in this chapter, with the individual patient.

LACK OF WILL OR LACK OF SKILL?

The heart and soul of quality in an audiology clinic is twofold: First, it rests with your ability to develop and implement a standardized process that is based on evidence-based-practice principles and best practice standards and, second, your ability to measure outcome in a comprehensive manner and use the data collected from patient outcome questionnaires to continually hone your standardized process. An inability to perform these two essential roles within your clinic usually comes down to two things: Either you need additional training in order to develop the skills to conduct these procedures with competence and confidence, or you lack the desire to gain the discipline needed to change ineffective habits and perform the procedures supported by the current best practice standards. Ultimately, the choice is yours.

REFERENCES

Abrams, H., Chisolm, T. H., McManus, M., & McArdle, R. (2012). Initial-fit versus verified prescription: Comparing self-perceived hearing aid benefit. *Journal of the American Academy of Audiology, 23*(10), 768–778.

Beck, D. L., & Harvey, M. A. (2009). Creating successful professional–patient relationships. *Audiology Today, September–October.*

Charles, C., Gafni A., & Whelan, T. (1997). Shared decision-making in the medical encounter: What does it mean? (Or it takes at least two to tango). *Social Science Medicine, 44*(5), 681–692.

Cox, R., & Alexander, G. (2007). Personality, hearing problems, and amplification characteristics: Contributions to self-report hearing aid outcomes. *Ear and Hearing, 28*(2), 141–162.

Davis, A., & Smith, P. (2008). Measuring quality in audiology, a global framework. *Audiology Today, 20*(6), 27–31.

Duhigg, C. (2012). *The power of habit.* New York, NY: Random House.

Gatehouse, S. (1994). Components and determinants of hearing aid benefit. *Ear and Hearing, 15*(1), 30–49.

Gopinath, B., Schneider, J., Hartley, D., Teber, D., McMahon, C. M., Leeder, S. R., & Mitchell, P. (2011). Incidence and predictors of hearing-aid use and ownership in older adults with hearing loss. *Annals of Epidemiology, 21*(7), 497–506.

Hartley, D., Rochtchina, E., Newall, P., Golding, M., & Mitchell, P. (2010). Use of hearing aids and assistive devices in an older Australian population. *Journal of the American Academy of Audiology, 21*, 642–653.

Harvey, M. A. (2001). *Listen with the heart: Relationships and hearing loss.* San Diego, CA: Dawnsign Press.

Kochkin, S. (2010). MarkeTrak VIII: Customer satisfaction with hearing aids is slowly increasing. *Hearing Journal, 63*(1), 11–19.

Kochkin, S. (2011). MarkeTrak VIII: Reducing patient visits through verification and validation. *Hearing Review, 18*(6), 10–12.

Kochkin, S., Beck, D. L., Christensen, L. A., Compton-Conley, C., Fligor, B. J., Kricos, P. B., . . . Turner, R. G. (2010). MarkeTrak VIII: The impact of the hearing healthcare professional on hearing aid user success. *Hearing Review, 17*(4), 12–34.

Miller, W. R., & Rollnick, S. (2002). *Motivational interviewing: Preparing people for change* (2nd ed.). New York, NY: Guilford Press.

Northern, J., & Beyer, C. M. (1999). Reducing hearing aid returns through patient education. *Audiology Today, 11*(2).

Saunders, G., & Forsline, A. (2012). Hearing-aid counseling: Comparison of single session informational counseling with single session performance-perceptual counseling. *International Journal of Audiology, 51*, 754–764.

Saunders, G. H. (2012). 20Q: Auditory training—Does it really work? *Audiology Online.* Retrieved from http://www.audiologyonline.com

Taylor, B., & Bernstein, J. (2011). The red flag matrix. *Audiology Practices, 3*(3), 40–51.

Walden, B., Demorest, M., & Helper, E. L. (1984). Self-report approach to assessing benefit derived from amplification. *Journal of Speech and Hearing Research, 27*, 49–56.

4

QUALITY IN ACTION AT THE FRONT DESK

A cornerstone of quality is that everyone in the organization is responsible for incrementally improving it. This chapter reinforces the fact that in any organization quality is the responsibility of everyone, including the front office professionals of an audiology practice. Using many of the concepts reviewed previously, this chapter demonstrates how quality can be brought to life in a practice by nonaudiologists who often have the role of providing front office support. Similar to how the best restaurants and the most effective hearing aid manufacturers operate, the most proficient front office professionals in hearing aid dispensing practices follow a regimented process with six distinct steps, which are outlined in this chapter. Although these six steps can be implemented throughout any organization, we examine how they are implemented with the front office personnel of a dispensing practice.

The information provided in this chapter is intended to be used by front office professionals of an audiology practice. In fact, you could use this chapter as a training manual for your front office staff, as it goes into considerable detail on *how* specific actions can be completed. Although the person behind the desk often goes by many names, such as receptionist, patient care coordinator, and front office professional (FOP), we stick with the latter name, as the term "front office professional" seems to be the most descriptive term for this critical role with any thriving clinic. In many ways the FOP is the most important person in your practice. This is especially true if you believe that first impressions are the most lasting ones. Considering that the FOP is usually the first voice that patients hear when calling your office, or the first friendly face they see when they enter the door, it is imperative for the FOP to be involved in any quality initiatives you are spearheading in your practice. Sadly, there is very little instructional material written for FOPs who are working in an audiology practice. Regardless of the role, here are the five steps, based on the concepts discussed in the first two chapters, that are needed to bring quality to life in a clinical practice:

1. Create a culture dedicated to excellence.
2. Hire well and orchestrate staff (division of labor).
3. Create and follow best practice standards.
4. Act on lead measures by providing feedback and coaching.
5. Update and incrementally improve performance and outcomes.

Let us review each of the aforementioned components through the lens of the FOP in a thriving hearing aid dispensing practice by first examining the critical role office culture plays.

CREATE A CULTURE DEDICATED TO EXCELLENCE

Culture is a term that has several meanings. For example, there are differences in culture between Americans and British just as there are between Bahamians and Australians. As nations have cultures, offices have them too. We briefly discussed culture in Chapter 1, and the important thing to remember is that culture is defined by the people who work in the office with the leader (likely to be you) setting the tone. As you know, a culture is any custom, more, and code of conduct that is considered acceptable behavior by the majority of the group. As the leader of your office it is largely up to you to establish this code of conduct. Things such as personal appearance are largely determined by the culture of the office. It might seem obvious, but you (assuming you are the leader or manager) establish your culture largely through your behaviors and values. By being on time, dressing appropriately, and acting in a professional manner, you are setting the tone for how you expect others in your culture to act.

If you aspire to run a practice that is known for quality, you will need to spend some time creating a culture that is consistent with this vision. You may remember in Chapter 1 we discussed the importance of having a vision for your practice. A vision is how you want others (namely the marketplace) to view you. Asking the simple question, "What do you want to be known for?" helps uncover your personal vision for your practice or career. Most professionals have a vision and want to create a culture around quality and excellence.

Also recall from Chapter 1 the importance of staging a memorable patient experience around six distinct "touch points" or interaction stations. Your culture serves as the focal point for many of the details of how you design and implement the patient experience in your practice. For example, you may choose to design a patient experience around optimizing your patients' personal relationships with family and friends through improved hearing and communication. In addition to "theming" your practice around a highly personalize experience (see Chapter 1 for more on the concept of "theming"), it is essential that your culture be representative of that same theme. In order to create an office culture that is congruent with your delivery of a memorable patient experience focusing on improved personal relationships, you need to strive to have a tight-knit group of staff that can deliver on your mission. Having weekly chat sessions, a morning devoted to coffee and donuts for the entire staff, or a monthly potluck lot may seem trivial, but orchestrating these events on a routine basis helps build your culture around your practice's theme. Regardless of exactly what you may do to build your culture, it is important that it center around the theme of the patient experience you are trying to provide. Table 4–1 shows some examples of themes and the underlying culture needed to foster a theme.

Table 4–1. Examples of Practice Themes and the Office Culture Needed to Support Them

If your theme is best described as . . .	Then the culture needed to support it is . . .
Family friendly	Warm and inviting
Traditionally medically oriented	Formal and businesslike
Centered around entertainment (e.g., musicals, old cars)	Relaxing

HIRE WELL AND ORCHESTRATE STAFF (DIVISION OF LABOR)

One of the most important things you will do in your practice is hire the right person to work as an FOP. Since almost every patient will come into contact with the FOP either over the phone or in person, the FOP must have impeccable interpersonal communication skills. In addition to being a warm and engaging person, the FOP must be a highly organized person with considerable attention to detail. In smaller practices you are likely to lean on one person to not only schedule appointments but to complete other necessary tasks, such as billing insurance and sending out letters to patients, among other common duties.

A lot of effort goes into making a hiring decision, but the primary consideration is the development of a comprehensive job description. The purpose of the job description is to thoroughly describe not only the duties of the position, but the experience requirements and skills needed to competently perform the job. Creating a job description goes beyond the scope of this chapter (there are several employee and human resource services that can help you create job descriptions); however, the main point from a quality perspective is that the job description is necessary in order to define the responsibilities of the FOP position. This requires that you spend some time thinking about the necessary skills and experience needed to conduct the fundamental behaviors outlined in the next section.

There are two other important aspects of the job description, especially as it relates to the front office professional. A good job description allows you to focus on the division of labor within your practice. Division of labor within a practice is deciding the specific tasks each staff member will conduct on a routine basis. For example, in a large audiology practice, it is important to identify the behaviors that generate the most revenue and reserve them for the licensed professional, who is typically the audiologist. Other important support tasks can then be identified and reserved for the FOP. Granted, there are many components involved in the division of labor and its financial impact on the practice, but from a quality perspective having a good idea of how you will divide labor in your practice is critical because it helps clearly define the roles of the staff and how

---

#DISCOVER

Once you know you can afford to hire another person, you need to carefully decide how this new staff member will contribute to the profitability of your business. Generally, there are three ways to divide your labor force (as characterized by Bob Wabler, former president of Amplifon USA):

- Staff who bring more patients to your practice through marketing. These are the "finders" within your practice.
- Staff who take care of the patients through consultative selling and clinical efforts. These are the "minders" in your practice.
- Staff who take care of the essential back office activities, such as phone scheduling, billing, and coding. These are the "grinders" in your practice.

Of course, in many practices the same person may play all three "finder–minder–grinder" roles simultaneously. Also, there are certainly times when you may want to contract an outside agency or consultant for special projects or assignments.

they fit together. Another reason for creating a comprehensive job description is that it forms the foundation for setting expectations. When a job description thoroughly describes all of the essential duties of a position, it reduces the chance that the wrong person will be hired for the job and it sets clear expectations from the beginning.

CREATE AND FOLLOW BEST PRACTICE STANDARDS

In this section we talk a lot about "behaviors" needed by the FOP in order to complete specific tasks. To some people the word "behavior" conjures up memories of disruptiveness in the classroom or poor conduct by a fellow employee. From a quality perspective behavior is not a negative word. Using the vernacular of quality, a behavior is simply the act of doing something, usually the interaction between patients and staff. In other words, virtually everything we do on the job is classified as a behavior. Another way to think about behavior is to contrast it with another important activity, which is thinking. Thinking does not require any action. Behaviors, on the other hand, are our thoughts put into action. Behavior is the act of doing something, and quality is the act of doing something in the most effective way that we can execute the behaviors. From a quality perspective, behaviors (or actions) are the assembly line of production. If you are building hearing aids, for example, all of the necessary steps required in the manufacturing process have been fine-tuned based on data collection and analysis relative to results. Through this process, the managers of the hearing aid assembly line, using data, have identified all of the actions that might result in defects to their product. Specific tasks that contribute to a reduction in variances of the assembly process that may result in a product defect become systematized. This same technique can be used in the identification of the behaviors to create best practices on the front lines of your practice. It is a series of behaviors (or actions) that are needed to create a successful hearing aid fitting and satisfied patient. For that reason, we focus on benchmarking a series of behaviors (or actions) that are likely to result in a satisfactory outcome and systematically improving them over time.

Another word often substituted for behaviors is "standards." A standard is best described as a "best practice behavior." A standard is a series of specific actions that are likely to result in repeatable outcomes. Let us get into some of the details of standards (or behaviors) that you might implement in your practice for FOPs. Note that the more specifically you can define the standards, the more likely you will be able to manage and coach effectively. Along with specific standards, you will need to create a few metrics that allow you to measure performance over time. Measuring performance over time will allow you to more effectively develop the skills of your FOP. (The following is an example of standards for an FOP for the second stage of the patient experience. See Figure 1–1 for details.)

The following section is written from the FOP's vantage point. As a general rule, it is the primary responsibility of the front office staff to efficiently and consistently schedule appointments. To keep your business running smoothly there is no duty that is more important than this one; therefore, to be successful in your position, you must master a question-and-answer process over the phone that is designed to lead the patient to the decision to make and keep an appointment.

A medically oriented business relies on patients coming through your doors on a consistent basis. Although marketing and advertising are important, the success of the practice largely rests on the ability of the FOP to book appointments effectively. This process of booking appointments starts with not only understanding your important role within the business, but how to conduct this process with skill and efficiency. As the old saying goes, it is much easier to get from point A to point B by following a straight line. The same is true when it comes to handling incoming and outgoing calls to and from customers.

It can be very easy to get off-track if you do not have a specific path to follow that leads to an appointment being made; therefore, it is your job to maintain control of the conversation when talking with patients over the phone. You must avoid, at all costs, *detailed* discussions about pricing, technology, insurance coverage, and the need for a hearing aid. These are all questions that should only be answered once the person comes for an appointment.

It seems like just about everyone complains about the quality of service they receive over the telephone. If you are lucky to actually talk to a live voice, that service representative is likely to be residing in a location that is several time zones away. Answering the phone effectively is a skill that can differentiate your practice. However, it just doesn't happen. Like everything, personalized telephone service requires planning, training and managerial oversight. Since booking appointments over the phone is probably the most pivotal role of the front office professional, let us review a detailed process for handling phone calls.

Five-Step Phone Scheduling Process

To help you stay on track, the protocol for scheduling an appointment has been broken down into five easy steps. These steps are designed not only to increase the number of appointments that you book, but are also critical to providing optimal customer service. These five steps are:

1. Greeting: sounding pleasant and upbeat when you answer the phone or personally greet a patient upon arrival in your office
2. Assessing the patient's wants and needs: the ability to discover the needs of the patient without sounding pushy or aggressive
3. Advising: the ability to answer questions succinctly using nontechnical language
4. Gaining agreement: the ability to schedule an appointment in a seamless manner
5. Thanking: the act of telling someone you appreciate their considerations and time

If you are the office manager, you may already know that regardless of the specific mission and theme that drive your practice, you need to ensure that the following expectations are established with your staff:

- They must perform their duties at the level the owner or manager expects.
- The company must be operated in a successful manner and strive to deliver on its promise of high-quality products and services.
- The patient who has come to you for help receives the most remarkable experience possible.
- You and the staff work together to identify gaps in service delivery and work together to improve those gaps.

Below is an example of how to deliver a remarkable service experience from the perspective of the FOP.

Step 1: Greeting

The standard phone greeting comprises these four core expectations:

1. All phones *must* be answered on or before the third ring.
2. All customers *must* be acknowledged within 30 seconds of entering your location. You can easily do this by making eye contact or with a small gesture.
3. Do not allow a call to rollover to the answering machine. Most customers will *not* leave a message—they may simply call your competition!
4. Keep your answering machine message up to date. Check it periodically to make sure it is working properly.

Standardized Greeting

The role of the manager is to ensure that all FOPs in the practice know the standard greeting. However, it is not enough to simply recite the greeting; FOPs must also know and understand the manner in which you want the greeting delivered. All phones must be answered using a standardized greeting. This is an example of a typical standardized greeting you could use in your practice:

> "Hello (Good Morning, Good Evening, Happy Holidays, etc.), thank you for calling (practice name). This is (Your First Name). How may I help you today?"

Of course, it is never as simple as robotically reciting a standardized greeting. It must sound authentic and natural. Keep in mind that *voice quality* is composed of the following components:

1. Tone (expresses feeling or emotion)
2. Inflection (emphasizes words and syllables to enhance a message)
3. Pitch (how high or how deep a voice is)
4. Rate (how many words are spoken per minute)
5. Volume (how loud or soft a voice sounds).

Often your voice quality is more important than the words you use. Mehrabian and Weiner (1967) published a seminal work on the components of communication. They were able to break down the components of communication and assign a percentage to how much each of the components contribute to the overall message. Since that time Albert Mehrabian has published several additional studies and books on communication. Perhaps his most popular work is the book *Silent Messages*. Mehrabian and colleagues have broken effective communication down into the following components:

Face-to-face communication:

- 55% body language
- 38% tone of voice
- 7% words used

Telephone communication:

- 82% tone of voice
- 18% words used

The lesson for FOPs is that most of your message is conveyed through tone of voice when talking over the phone; thus, it is important that you spend time developing a pleasant voice. Mehrabian and Wiener's (1967) work suggests that how you sound is more important that what you actually say. Obviously, the FOP must be able to accurately answer questions over the phone, but time needs to be spent ensuring that the FOPs voice sounds pleasant and helpful. When it comes to verbal commu-

---

#DISCOVER

Mystery Shopping

In some situations, it is helpful to use objective information in the standardization and coaching process. There are several companies that offer mystery shopping services. These services record the dialogue between a representative of the mystery shopping service and the FOP. They may even record calls between patients and employees. These services provide a recording of that dialogue to the manager who can use it for coaching purposes. Before using any mystery shopping program, it is important to check with your state and local employee privacy laws. It is also best practice to inform your employees that you may record their calls.

---

nication both over the phone and in-person, we know people should never speak more than 160 to 180 words per minute. To check your rate of speech, choose a passage from your favorite magazine and record yourself reading it for 1 minute. Then count the number of words you read. Do this exercise three times with three different passages.

When speaking to your patients, remember these tips:

1. You *must* speak clearly and your voice should convey warmth. *Smile* when you speak. Even if you are not in a good mood, you must *always* make the patient feel special and that you personally care about him/her.
2. Refer to the patient as Mr./Mrs./Ms. unless the patient gives you permission to use his/her first name.
3. Be authentic and empathic. Somebody once said that priests are the psychologists of the poor, and the same can be said of audiologists and their relationship to adults with hearing loss. Elderly people often seek our services and want to unload their emotional burden of coping with hearing loss for several years. They come to discuss something very personal—their hearing—and they would like to have a

sympathetic ear when they do so. Use phrases like, "We are here to help." Or, "I understand what you mean."

4. Avoid the use of jargon (vocabulary specific to a particular trade or profession), slang (the informal use of words that are characteristically more vivid and playful than ordinary language), and quirks (poor grammar, irritating sounds, strange expressions).

5. The role of a manager is to provide feedback and coaching on any phone behavior that is distracting and ineffective. In a culture of continuous improvement, everyone must be striving to find ways to incrementally enhance the service delivery experience.

It is also important that managers have a process in place for how callers are placed on hold. You cannot assume that someone knows the best practice for conducting this process. Below are best practice behaviors for placing a call on hold.

Putting a Caller on Hold

If you are on another line or talking to a patient in-person when a call comes in, follow this process:

1. Politely excuse yourself or ask permission to put the caller on hold.

2. Greet the other caller by saying:

   "Hello. Thank you for calling (your practice's name). Your call is very important to me but I am currently on the other line. Do you mind being placed on hold?" (Wait until the patient gives you permission!)"

3. If you discover that you are going to take longer than 30 seconds to get back to the patient, ask for his/her phone number and call them back at a specified time. Make sure you get the patient's permission to do this.

Step 2: Assessing Patient Needs

The second step of the phone scheduling stage of the patient experience is the ability to efficiently assess the needs of a patient. Use open-ended questions (questions that begin with who, what, when, where, why, how, or tell me) to discover what the patient needs. He/she may not always tell you everything you need to know. The trick is that you must ask these questions while at the same time answering any questions the patient may have.

There are five questions that are listed below that are critical to ask. Not only do they provide information the provider needs, but they can also help in determining the type of appointment you schedule, while letting the patient know that you care about his/her hearing health.

Rather than using a script, you can formulate your own series of needs-assessment questions around the five provided below. By asking this series of questions you will begin to uncover the need of the patient and move toward scheduling an appointment (assuming that is why the patient is calling):

1. For whom is the appointment?
2. What, if any, irritation, discomfort, or pain are you (or your family member) experiencing in your ears?
3. When was the last time you (family member) had your (his/her) hearing tested?
4. Describe any problems you (or your family member) may have when communicating with others.
5. When would you like to come in for an appointment?

These questions can be asked as part of the normal conversation or, if you first ask the patient's permission, you can ask these questions all at once: "Mr. Smith, I have a few questions that we ask all our patients prior to scheduling an appointment. It helps us better understand what might be happening prior to the visit. Do you mind if I ask those questions now?"

Answering Frequently Asked Questions

If possible, try to answer all the patient's questions within 15 seconds or less from the start of the phone call. There are several topics that are universally required to have a well-thought answer. The following questions are some of the most common asked of the FOP. Each of these questions require a precise,

---

#DISCOVER

Answering the Phone with a Pleasant Voice

Since vocal inflection is such a significant part of communication over the phone, the proper vocal intonation is even more important than a script. One of the universal rules of communication is that your initial greeting sets the tone for the entire conversation. Listeners tend to mirror the emotions of the speaker. For example, if you are agitated when you make a call to a customer service desk, and the receptionist answers the phone with a pleasant demeanor, it is extremely difficult to stay agitated throughout the entire conversation.

---

semiscripted answer. Managers need to work with FOPs to craft the responses that best reflect the values and mission of your practice, of course, but here are some examples:

1. *What makes your practice different from the competition?* Our practice has been in the area for more than 30 years and we are quite proud of our reputation. Dr. Taylor has successfully worked with thousands of patients and his entire staff is dedicated to providing the most thorough patient experience you can imagine. We are known for delivering comprehensive care.

2. *How much do hearing aids cost?* Hearing aids in this office range from $2,000 to $6,000 per pair. The cost depends on the size and style of the hearing aid and also the type of technology. With modern hearing aids, the customer has numerous choices; therefore, it is important to discuss all the possibilities with Dr. Taylor. Because we offer customized care, our prices reflect that service.

3. *How do I know which hearing aid is best for me?* You must first have your hearing examined by Dr. Taylor to determine if you are even a candidate for hearing aids. Once the need for hearing aids has been established, Dr. Taylor may pro-

pose various styles, makes, and technologies based on your specific communication needs. In addition to the devices, we offer several types of services that may be appropriate for you.

4. *What is the process for getting a hearing aid?* Prior to being fitted with hearing aids, it is very important to be examined to determine the extent and type of hearing loss you have. Following that, Dr. Taylor will explain the test findings in detail and determine if you are a candidate for hearing aids. If you are a candidate for hearing aids, Dr. Taylor will recommend the type of amplification that would be appropriate for your hearing loss and lifestyle.

5. *What if I don't like them? Does your office offer a trial period?* This office offers a 45-day evaluation period on all devices. During that period, Dr. Taylor will ensure that you are receiving the maximum benefit from your hearing aids.

6. *Do you repair hearing aids?* Our staff can check your hearing aid and determine if the problem is something they can repair in our office or whether it requires factory service. If your device must be sent to the factory or manufacturer, the repair cost will be about $500 and that will include a 12-month warranty.

7. *Do hearing aids use batteries?* All hearing aids use batteries. They are easy to change yourself. Depending on the style and type, most batteries last 1 to 4 weeks and will cost you a couple of dollars per month.

8. *Do you charge for a hearing examination? If so, what is the cost?* Yes, we charge for hearing examinations. The fee for the evaluation is $100. We can check to see if your insurance provider will reimburse for that service.

9. *Does insurance cover the cost of hearing aids?* Many major insurance companies do not provide hearing aid benefits; however, there are increasingly more managed care operations that have negotiated hearing aid benefits from certain providers. Those insurance programs that have a hearing aid benefit are typically union-negotiated contracts for employees who may be at risk for hearing loss from occupational noise. I would be happy to get your insurance information and contact your company to determine what, if any, benefits you have.

Step 3: Advising

The next step involves moving from questioning to advising. During this step of the phone conversation you should focus on emphasizing the benefits of an appointment. This requires the FOP to communicate the benefits and end results of an appointment, rather than what happens during the appointment. This three-step exercise is designed to help the FOP keep the end in mind and focus on the patient benefits of a scheduled appointment. The exercise will help the FOP uncover the patient's benefit of making an appointment by articulating answers that highlight end results:

1. List the features of a hearing aid consultation appointment: "Consultations with the audiologist do not take more than an hour, are painless, and are relatively inexpensive."
2. Ask yourself, "so what?" about the features you listed. Asking "so what?" allows you to determine the risk to the patient and how it can be addressed. A hearing aid consultation is needed to identify the extent of any hearing problem and customize a solution and level of service required to address the hearing problem.
3. Ask yourself, "What will scheduling a hearing aid consultation allow my patient to do?" The answer to this question is likely to be about how improved communication will result in better relationships with family, less stress, and an overall improved quality of life.

It is important to note that these questions are not asked directly to the patient; rather, you need to ask yourself these questions to ensure that you are addressing the concerns of the patient and translating that phone conversation into a scheduled appointment.

Another element of the advising stage of the booking process is remote rapport building. This means that you are not "selling" the patient on the virtues of the *device*, but on the professionalism and expertise of the staff. Interwoven throughout your conversation should be your ability to tout the virtues of the professionalism the patient is going to see. Keeping in mind the patient experience model outlined in Chapter 1, one of your primary roles is to make the audiologist or primary service provider the star of the show. Here is an example of what you can say to keep the audiologist in the starring role for the patient:

> "I am confident that you will love working with Dr. Taylor. He is very thorough and all our patients just adore him."

#DISCOVER

The acronym SOLERS is a reminder of some necessary behaviors that will help you communicate in a polished, professional, and authentic manner both on the phone and in-person. SOLERS is a term to remember when it comes to effective communication:

S: squarely face the customer (or an object that you can visualize in your office while on the phone)

O: open posture (do not cross your legs or arms)

L: lean forward slightly

E: eye contact

R: relax and take a deep breath or two

S: smile!

Step 4: Gaining Agreement

This is the step where you ask for the appointment. Use this script as a guide to transition from the last "needs-assessing" question to asking for the appointment.

> "Let's try to get some definitive answers to your questions by booking an appointment with Dr. Taylor. Consultations are free so you don't have to worry about any costs for a few minutes of his time. I have an opening at (___ AM/PM or ___ AM/PM). How does that sound?"

Here is a slightly different way to ask for the appointment:

> "The next step is to schedule a hearing evaluation appointment. I can go ahead and book the appointment now. What day next week is best for you to come in?"

Sometimes the patient does not agree to make an appointment right away. They will make an objection. Sometimes this objection is just a "stall" and not a real objection at all. In fact, the most common type of objection is nonthreatening requests for additional information. Remember, the patient will only agree to buy if they trust you and see value in setting the appointment. It is critical for the FOP to be adept at anticipating and addressing objections, especially ones that occur during phone calls. There are four steps to handling objections:

1. Listen: Do not anticipate what the patient is going to say. Stop talking and listen.
2. Restate: Repeat what the customer has said to ensure you understand what the objection is.
3. Ask: Ask the patient additional questions to help clarify the issue.
4. Answer: Nearly all objections can be answered with practice. Answers to common objections are listed below.

Common Objections

The following is a list of some of the most common objections to scheduling an appointment during a phone call. Along with the objection is some sample dialogue you can use to address it.

1. *I cannot afford a (new) hearing instrument.* I understand that price is an issue. It is a concern for everyone. Dr. Taylor's goal is to improve your quality of life. I know he will work with you to get the best devices that fit into your personal budget. How does that sound?

    I know you have made a tremendous investment in your current hearing aids. Since proper maintenance is critical in achieving the peak performance of your hearing aids, and since you have already invested so much in your existing aids, it makes sense to ensure they are well taken care of.

Let's book an appointment so we can clean them and test them to see if they are performing the way they should. Does this sound like a good idea to you?

2. *I have come back to this office several times and it has never been right.* I apologize for the inconvenience. I know it must be frustrating to have to come back all the time, especially when you have invested so much money in your new hearing aids.

   It is the policy of this office to work with all our customers until they are completely satisfied. Sometimes it takes a great deal of fine-tuning to ensure that your hearing aids fit properly and are accurately programmed to improve your ability to hear. Attention to detail is of utmost importance to us. In the end, your patience will be rewarded with improved hearing. Is there any way I can make coming to an appointment easier for you?

3. *I just purchased new hearing aids from someone else.* I am glad to hear that you made the decision to invest in your hearing health. How are they working for you? That's great. I want you to know that we still have your file and that you are welcome here any time. We would be more than happy to clean and service your hearing instruments for you.

4. *I lost my hearing aid.* I'm so sorry to hear that! Losing a hearing aid must have a negative affect on your lifestyle! How have you been functioning without it? Since it is time for your checkup anyway, I recommend that you schedule an appointment. Do Mondays or Tuesdays work better for you? When you come in, we will be able to determine what your options are.

5. *I am too busy to make an appointment right now.* I can understand that an active personal or work schedule can be hectic! Don't put off your hearing aid checkup too long, however; hearing aids require periodic maintenance. By focusing on protecting your investment with a regularly scheduled "clean and check," your hearing aids will continue to be in excellent working condition. Would it be all right if I called you next week to schedule an appointment? Is there a day or time you would like me to call?

6. *I do not drive and there is no one here to bring me into the office.* Since you do not have access to readily accessible

transportation, it sounds like we need to do a little advance planning to make arrangements for you to come into the office. Who normally takes you to the doctor or dentist's office? Do you think that person would be willing to bring you here so you can have your hearing evaluated? I would be glad to work with you to pick a time that would be convenient for both of you. Would you like me to call that person for you?

7. *I rarely wear my hearing aids. They do not need cleaning.* May I ask you a few questions? Why are you not wearing your hearing aids? Are they not comfortable? I recommend that we book an appointment for you to see if we can improve the fit (or sound quality). At that time, we will also take the opportunity to clean them. After all, it only takes a tiny piece of wax to have a negative effect on the ability of your hearing aids to work properly. What day works best for you, Monday or Tuesday?

8. *I hear just as well without my hearing aids.* You *should* notice a considerable difference when you use your hearing aids. If you hear as well without them, it could be because your hearing aids are not working properly. Let's schedule an appointment to see if they are plugged with wax, or if the battery contacts need cleaning. What day works best for you, Monday or Tuesday?

9. *I recently saw a doctor who said I do not need hearing aids.* I am glad to hear that you discuss your ability to hear with your doctor because too many people do not. It is possible that your doctor meant nothing could be done *medically* to restore your hearing. Although 90% of all hearing losses are not medically treatable, these hearing losses can be improved through the use of hearing aids. Have you ever had your hearing tested? A hearing evaluation is the first step in dealing with a loss of hearing. Let's schedule a time for you to come in to have an evaluation. At that time, you can have all your questions answered by (person's name). What day works best for you, Monday or Tuesday?

10. *I am too old/sick to bother with hearing aids.* It must be hard to be motivated to make appointments when you are not feeling well. But you must know you are very important to us. We want to make sure your hearing instruments are

working the way they should so you can enjoy the sounds around you. Is there a particular day of the week on which having an appointment would work for you? We can be very flexible and the appointment itself will not take very long. We would love to see you.

11. *Just send me some literature.* I would be glad to send you some literature. What is your name, address, and phone number? I will put some information in the mail today. Once you have read the material, you will be well informed and should have questions. Is it okay for me to call you 10 days from now to answer any questions you might have?

#DISCOVER

Brevity

There is no better way to lose a call than to give too much information. Excessively long and meandering answers confuse your customer and often sound contrived and insincere. Your responses should be brief and to the point. When in doubt, simply say that the hearing care professional in your clinic would love to provide a more detailed explanation, and that this requires the patient to make a personal visit to the clinic.

Patient Who Books an Appointment

Once a patient makes a decision to schedule an appointment, there are several things to consider during the booking process. These factors include:

1. Offering a choice of appointment times
2. Ensuring a family member or friend accompanies the customer to the appointment
3. Entering the customer's name, address, and phone number into the database system
4. Capturing lead source information (primary and secondary)
5. Gathering insurance information (if appropriate and necessary).

Customer Who Refuses to Book an Appointment

Occasionally, you will have a patient who refuses to schedule an appointment. In those cases the following process is recommended:

1. Offering to send information to every customer who chooses not to book an appointment
2. Entering the customer's name, address, and phone number into the database system
3. Capturing lead source information (primary and secondary).

#DISCOVER

Communicating with the Elderly

Many patients in a hearing aid dispensing practice are over the age of 80 years. Due to their advancing age, there are several issues that might make communication difficult for this group. In addition to a hearing loss, this group of patients may suffer from dementia and vision difficulties. Here are some tips for communicating with the elderly:

- Encourage them to use a telephone with visual captions. Oaktree products has several models from which to choose.
- Use E-mail communication.
- Slow down your rate of speech and rephrase when necessary.
- Ask to speak to a caregiver or member of the family.
- Be patient and understanding of their situation.

Friend or Family Member Attendance Request

A best practice behavior for scheduling appointments over the phone is the request for the patient to bring along a significant other. Follow this script to explain to the patient why he/she needs to bring a family member to the appointment:

> "Dr. Taylor requests that you bring someone with you for the evaluation, preferably your spouse or a significant other.

Would it be possible to bring a loved one or friend with you to the appointment?"

If the patient asks why this is needed, simply state that the audiologist knows that coping with hearing loss is something that affects family relationships and it is helpful to get some input from a significant other or family member.

As a rule of thumb, approximately 60 to 70% of all first-time patients coming in for a hearing evaluation should have a loved one attend the appointment. Managers should track this on a weekly basis.

Step 5: Thanking and Confirming

The final stage of the booking process is formally thanking the patient for the call. Do not forget this critical phase of the five-step selling process. Patients want to know that they are appreciated and that they made the right decision. Thank them for choosing you—even if they do not make an appointment!

1. Congratulate the patient for taking steps to improve their hearing health.
2. Reconfirm the day and time of the appointment prior to ending the call and tell the patient he/she will be reminded of his/her appointment.
3. Remind the patient to bring their insurance card or forms with him to the appointment.
4. Offer directions or offer to send a map to the patient. You may also share a link to your Web site.

@*CONNECT*

A Standardized Greeting

A cornerstone of quality is reducing variance in your product. A standard greeting, along with semiscripted answers to common questions, reduces variance. Von Hansen, a consultant to the hearing aid industry, has created an easy-to-use script for FOPs. Go to http://www.vonhanseninc.com for details.

Putting It All Together

The following sample dialogue incorporates the five-step selling protocol we have just reviewed. Critical elements of each step have been identified for your reference.

Incoming Call Script: Appointment Scheduled

The phone rings.

> *FOA:* Good morning. Thank you for calling Taylor Hearing Center. This is Mary. How may I help you today? (Standardized greeting)
>
> *Patient:* Hi. I heard your ad on the radio and I'm calling to find out how much hearing aids cost. Can you help?
>
> *FOA:* I most certainly can, Mr . . . What is your name?
>
> *Patient:* Bill Smith.
>
> *FOA:* Mr. Smith, hearing aids generally cost from a few hundred to a few thousand dollars depending on your unique needs. Who will be wearing the hearing aids?
>
> *Patient:* I'm calling for myself. I'm not ready to buy anything yet. I'm just curious about the cost. That range you gave me is rather broad. What is the difference between your low-price hearing aid and the one at the top of the price range?
>
> *FOA:* I understand . . . you are doing a little research. That's a wise decision since there are so many options available to you today. (Shows empathy) In general, the level of technology determines the price of the hearing aid. The more technologically advanced, the more expensive. What, if any, irritation, discomfort, or pain are you experiencing in your ears?
>
> *Patient:* I'm not experiencing any pain or discomfort, just a hearing loss that I've had for a while.
>
> *FOA:* Thanks for sharing that. It is helpful to know. (Shows that you are listening) Mr. Smith, when was the last time you had your hearing tested?

Patient: You can call me Bill. I believe I had my hearing tested about 3 years ago.

FOA: So Bill, do you currently wear one or two hearing aids?

Patient: I don't wear any hearing aids. I own a pair that I bought a couple of years ago, but they never seemed to work, so I don't wear them.

FOA: Sorry to hear that. Maybe we can take a look at those here in the clinic. Considering your hearing ability now, can you describe any problems you may have when communicating with others?

Patient: I've noticed that I've had to turn the volume up on the TV more frequently. That's why I dug out my old hearing aids, but like I said, they never did work.

FOA: Turning up the volume on the TV is a common indicator that someone could possibly be experiencing some level of hearing loss, although it could be something as simple as earwax build-up. Let's try to get some definitive answers to your questions by booking an appointment with Dr. Taylor. I have an opening at 9 AM or 2 PM next Tuesday. How does that sound?

Patient: Yes. But all I wanted to know is how much hearing aids cost. Can't you be a little more specific? I can't afford to spend too much.

FOA: We have many types of hearing aids so I am sure Dr. Taylor can accommodate your budget; however, to give you the professional answers you are looking for, we will need to evaluate your hearing first. I recommend that we go ahead and set up a time for you to talk with him.

Patient: Well, I guess that would be okay. How much will that cost?

FOA: The cost for an evaluation is $85. We can check to see if your insurance will pay all or part of that fee. Would you mind sharing your insurance details with me and I can check on that prior to your appointment?

Patient: That's okay, I will go ahead and make the appointment and give that to you when I am there.

FOA: Sounds good. So, may I ask, who can come with you to your appointment?

Patient: My wife will come with me.

FOA: Could you two come to the office next Tuesday?

Patient: That would work.

FOA: Great! Tuesday it is. What time is better for you, mornings or afternoons?

Patient: Afternoons before 3 PM.

FOA: How about Tuesday at 2 PM?

Patient: That's fine. Oh, I have one more question. Does insurance cover the cost of hearing aids?

FOA: Most major insurance companies do not provide hearing aid benefits; however, there are increasingly more managed care operations that have negotiated hearing aid benefits from certain providers. I would be happy to take your insurance information and contact your company to determine what, if any, benefits you have. Make sure you bring your insurance card with you. Do you know how to get to the office?

Patient: No, not really.

FOA: It's really easy to find. I will send you a map today. Bill, I want to sincerely thank you for calling us with questions about your ability to hear. You will be in great hands with Dr. Taylor. I will call and confirm your appointment 24 hours ahead of time and I look forward to meeting you and Mary next Wednesday at 2 PM. Bye now.

Patient: Good-bye.

Incoming Call Script: No Appointment Scheduled

Here is another example of the dialogue between a caller, who is himself not a potential patient but instead is enquiring about a relative who is, and the FOP. The teaching point of this sec-

> ### #DISCOVER
>
> ### How to Track Companion Attendance
>
> Effective managers know that, if they want to improve something, they must first begin to measure it. Considering the fact that the majority of our customers will not make a purchasing decision without input from their spouse or significant other, it is critical to the success of the business to monitor the number of customers arriving at the first appointment with a companion. Front office professionals must be trained on how to encourage prospects to bring their companion to the initial consultation appointment. As a general rule, 60 to 70% of all first-time consultation appointments should include a companion.

tion is that your standards and expectations must become part of the routine behavior of your staff in order to create a culture committed to excellence that results in high-quality outcomes.

The phone rings.

FOA: Good morning. Thank you for calling Taylor Hearing Services. This is Mary. How may I help you today? (Standardized greeting)

Caller: Hi. I'm visiting my Dad and I think he may have a hearing problem. Can you tell me a little bit about your clinic?

FOA: I most certainly can, Mr. . . . . What is your name?

Caller: Steve Jones.

FOA: Mr. Jones, Dr. Taylor has been in practice for more than 10 years and he offers a wide range of hearing services. Since our entire staff is so focused on listening to your needs and offering solutions, you can be confident that we will be there for you when you need a guarantee of support and follow-up.

You said your father might have a hearing problem. Do you mind if I ask you a few questions about that?

Caller: No, not at all.

FOA: Mr. Jones, what, if any, irritation, discomfort, or pain is he experiencing in his ears?

Caller: I am not aware that he is experiencing any pain.

FOA: Well, that's good. When was the last time he had his hearing tested?

Caller: I'm not sure. I know he has had it tested before, several years ago, and that he has some level of hearing loss, but he refused to wear hearing aids at that time.

FOA: So, he is not wearing any aids currently?

Caller: No, he never has.

FOA: Can you describe any problems he has when communicating with others?

Caller: I've noticed that he has to turn the volume up on the TV more frequently, and that if I talk to him when he is not looking at me, he doesn't respond.

FOA: Turning up the volume on the TV and not responding to conversation are common indicators that someone could possibly be experiencing some level of hearing loss, although it could be something as simple as earwax build-up. Let's get some definitive answers to your questions by booking an appointment with Dr. Taylor. I have an opening next week in the morning and afternoon. How does that sound?

Caller: I would have to talk to my father first, so I'm not going to be able to book an appointment at this time. And I know he's not going to want to come in. He just doesn't think he has a hearing problem.

FOA: It sounds like he might be in some denial, which is not uncommon. May I recommend something?

Caller: Sure.

FOA: If you go to our Web site, you can take an online questionnaire that shows how much hearing loss might be affecting him and your family. Here's the Web site . . .

http://www.taylorhearing.com. Look for the yellow hearing screening questionnaire at the top left. If the Internet is handy, I can walk you through it while you are on the phone with me right now.

Caller: That's ok. Let me talk to him, and if I have any luck I'll call you back.

FOA: Great. In the meantime, why don't you give me your address and phone number so I can send you some literature about coping with hearing loss?

Caller: (Gives address and phone number)

FOA: Thank you. I will put the information in the mail today. Mr. Jones, I want to sincerely thank you for calling us with questions about your father's hearing health. Everyone here really appreciates that you gave us the opportunity to help you. I look forward to meeting you and your father soon. Thanks again. Bye now.

Caller: You've been very helpful. Good-bye.

In addition to the specific behaviors listed here, it is helpful to post the customer service standards of your office for staff to see. Recall from Chapters 1 and 2 that checklists can be used to communicate standards and best practices. Once FOPs have been hired and oriented to your office culture, it is the responsibility of the manager to instill your office standards. Below is an example of quality-of-care standards you may have for the FOP in your practice.

ACT ON LEAD MEASURES BY PROVIDING FEEDBACK AND COACHING

Once standards and their underlying behaviors have been established, it is imperative that the manager or owner routinely evaluate and inspect the standards. Although the word "inspect" might sound a little over-the-top, it accurately describes the process of ensuring that expectations are being met. In the parlance of clinical audiology, the act of inspection of your standards is similar to verifying a prescriptive gain target using probe-microphone measures. The prescription target (e.g., NAL-NL2) is the standard, the behaviors are your ability to conduct the probe-microphone measure, and the act of inspection is your ability to see how closely the probe microphone responses match the prescribed fitting targets.

The two core components involved in taking action on lead measures are the use of a scorecard and the ability to deliver effective feedback to staff. In the case of the FOP it is important to measure his or her ability to conduct their key responsibilities, which are scheduling appointments and greeting patients. In order to measure these competencies, you need to use a combination of objective or proxy measures. (Recall the proxy measures discussed in Chapter 2.) Proxy measures enable the manager to ascertain whether an important task was completed by observing other behaviors or actions related to the important task.

Perhaps the most important direct measure of productivity is daily tracking of phone calls answered and appointments scheduled. This is shown in Table 4–2. It is also helpful to measure the companion-attendance ratio for all new appointments.

Table 4–2. Hypothetical comparison of results for two hearing aid dispensing offices with the same operational variables. The key difference between these two offices is the quality of the front office professional.

Activity	Office 1 (Ineffective)	Office 2 (Effective)
Calls per day	12	12
Appointments made per day	1	6
Appointments made per week	5	30
Patients purchasing hearing aids	2	12
Number of units sold	3	21
Revenue generated	$6,000	$42,000

Proxy measures of quality are needed in order to evaluate and continuously improve the behaviors associated with service delivery. Since the core behaviors associated with the FOP's work are related to communication skills over the phone and in-person, a checklist or scorecard can be used to benchmark and incrementally improve gaps in performance. Adapting many of Six Sigma-like techniques enables you to benchmark best practice behaviors, identify gaps, and then develop a plan to improve them over time.

Table 4–3 shows an example of a scorecard that can be used by the manager to evaluate and monitor best practice behaviors associated with FOP duties. After the FOP has been properly trained and working for a few months, the manager may begin the process of periodic evaluation. In the spirit of maintaining an office culture devoted to excellence, it is imperative that the FOP understand that you are not micromanaging them. By clearly communicating on a constant basis that best practice standards, measurement, and continuous improvement are an integral part of your office culture, you are more likely to get the buy-in of the staff.

The fundamental behaviors shown in column one of Table 4–3 are the necessary skills needed to optimize performance. If the manager observes that a fundamental behavior is being conducted properly, an "X" is placed in the proper column. The

Table 4–3. Front Office Professional Scorecard

Fundamental Behavior	Satisfactory	Needs Development
Phone greeting		
In-person greeting		
Questions over the phone		
Advising over the phone		
Asking for the appointment		
Thanking		

choice of words is very deliberate. In a culture devoted to continuous improvement, employees should be encouraged to always be developing a new skill or fine-tuning an existing one. Framing self-improvement as development helps to eliminate defensive behavior when a skill has been judged as needing work. If a fundamental behavior does need work, a summary of how the behavior falls short of expectations is noted in the "needs development" column. It is the responsibility of the manager to ensure that each FOP understands how to complete these fundamental behaviors on a routine basis. Once that process is complete, the manager is responsible for ensuring that any observable or measureable gaps are eliminated through coaching.

UPDATE AND INCREMENTALLY IMPROVE PERFORMANCE AND OUTCOMES

Once you have implemented a scorecard like the one shown in Table 4–4, it is necessary to have a mechanism in place that allows you to help the FOP continually fine-tune their skills. There are two mechanisms that allow you to improve gaps in performance and the fundamental behaviors that drive that performance: providing direct feedback and coaching. Feedback and coaching complement one another. They are intended to raise awareness about any performance gaps and eliminate them. Feedback is the act of verbally communicating to staff in a nonthreatening manner on a regular basis how the FOP is conducting their job in relation to your standards. The goal of feedback is to provide the FOP with information with respect to their performance so that they can improve. The key to delivering feedback is to establish a culture of inclusiveness and continuous self-improvement. In addition, feedback must be delivered on a daily basis and most of it should be of a positive nature. The essence of providing feedback is that it allows staff to know where they stand with respect to expectations and performance. There is a systematic process you can use to deliver feedback. To deliver positive feedback, which reinforces your standards and culture, do the following:

Table 4–4. A Sample Front Office Professional Scorecard

Skill	Demonstrated Proficiency	Action Item
Set-up and ready to go at the start of the business day		
Pleasant sounding voice		
Ability to consistently (<50% of calls) book appointment with new prospects		
Ability to Listen Intently and Answer Patient Questions		
Friendly Personal Greeting Upon Patient Arrival		
Show Empathy to Patients		
Complete Patient Paperwork Accurately and Timely (Billing and Coding)		

Step 1: Get permission from the FOP to share information. "Can I share something with you, Bonnie?"

Step 2: Manager says: "When you (restate the specific action performed by the FOP) it does (consequences of the action)" Example: "When you went out to the parking lot to help that patient into the car, I could see how happy his wife was while she waited in the front seat."

Step 3: Manager praises: "Great job!"

#DISCOVER

Attitude Versus Behavior

This chapter goes into a lot of detail on FOP behavior. Unlike attitude, which cannot be observed, behaviors are readily observed and often reflect an underlying attitude. Since behaviors can be observed and measured, they form the foundation of quality from the perspective of the FOP.

Positive feedback for even the smallest actions can go a long way in building a culture of inclusiveness and excellence. On the other hand, another type of feedback called self-improvement feedback—when delivered with empathy and understanding—can help close gaps in performance. Self-improvement feedback needs to be delivered when a behavior is limiting performance or affecting the quality of care.

Step 1: Get permission from the FOP to share information. "Can I share something with you, Bonnie?"

Step 2: Manager says: "When you do (restate the specific action performed by the FOP) it does (consequences of the action)" Example: "When you come in 15 minutes late, it puts everyone in an awkward position. I noticed that we had a patient sitting in the waiting room without being helped."

Step 3: Ask the employee what they can do differently to improve or what is needed for them to improve. Example: "How can I help with this situation?"

The feedback model presented here might sound harsh and aggressive. The critical part of communicating expectations through this feedback model is that it must be delivered in a kind and respectful manner. When you have established a culture based on a commitment to excellence, set clear standards, delivered adequate training, and provided constant positive feedback, the self-improvement feedback that managers need to deliver with candor will be communicated much easier than you may think.

@*CONNECT*

To learn more about other behaviorally based management techniques visit http://www.manager-tools.com/.

In addition to providing feedback on a regular basis, the
manager must identify gaps in performance that require coaching.
Although managers can work together with the FOP to identify
areas in performance that need to be improved, coaching is usually
a task that can be outsourced. There are numerous adult education centers, community colleges, and websites that offer courses
on phone rapport, communication strategies, as well as billing
and coding—all tasks that many FOPs are expected to perform.

Once a performance gap has been identified, the role of the
manager is to work with the FOP to put together an action plan
that results in improved performance. This action plan needs to
include specific areas of improvement, the actions that will be
taken to improve performance, and the time needed to improve
performance. An action plan like the one described here sounds
strict, but in a culture of continuous improvement where all staff
is looking to improve something, it becomes a cornerstone of
quality. This chapter lays the groundwork for establishing quality
in the front office of an audiology practice. Using the concepts
established in the first two chapters, you can build quality into
your organization by implementing the processes discussed in
this chapter. In the end, a good process pleases the people who
use it, enhances their ability to do more, creates value for the
organization, and, ultimately, improves quality of care for patients.

CUSTOMER SERVICE STANDARDS

The following customer service standards are strongly recommended:

1. Answer the phone on or before the third ring. Acknowledge
   the customer within 30 seconds of the time he or she enters
   the location.

2. Determine the wants and needs of the customer.
3. Stress the benefits of an appointment and/or services.
4. Recommend that the customer bring a companion to the appointment.
5. Overcome any objections to ensure an appointment is made.
6. Thank the customer and gather insurance information (if applicable).

Make multiple copies of the Customer Service Standards and place one by all the phones in the office. This will remind staff of the actions needed to create a culture of excellence that results in high-quality outcomes for patients.

#DISCOVER

The RATER Model

Instill the essential behaviors by training your FOP to follow the RATER model. RATER is an acronym that can help you know the steps to effective communication over the phone:

Reliability—timeliness/consistency/accuracy

Assurance—respect/credibility/confidentiality

Tangibles—answer questions about hearing aid technology

Empathy—transparency/clear communication/personalize

Responsiveness—prompt attention/flexibility/complaint handling.

The previous section was devoted to the standards and expected behavior of the FOP in regards to scheduling appointments. There are at least two other key skills that are a necessary part of the FOA's job in a hearing aid dispensing practice.

GREETING PATIENTS AND PUTTING THEM AT EASE

In an audiology practice you often work directly with clientele that is nervous and apprehensive about their inability to hear. Of course, this is a natural by-product of hearing loss of adult onset. An important role of the FOP is to recognize some of the normal behaviors of an adult with gradual hearing loss, such as denial, avoidance, and even hostility, and have some communication strategies to put patients at ease about their appointment.

Taking the time to fine-tune the details of how the FOP should greet a patient upon arrival is critical to any culture. When a patient arrives in your office, they should be greeted as if he or she were a well-respected Hollywood actor or a member of the British royal family. In addition to proper eye contact, the FOP needs to stand up and acknowledge the patient at the check-in desk. Smiling and shaking their hand are other components of a competent greeting. The final stages of the in-person greeting should comprise providing a warm verbal greeting, asking the patient to provide any information, such as insurance card, and guiding the patient to a seat in the reception area. It also helps to advise the patient of activities they can do in the reception area and about how long they may have to wait to see the audiologist. Of course, when patients have been waiting more than about 15 minutes, the FOP needs to personally check with the patient to see if anything is needed. In short, patients need to be greeted in your practice like you would greet a good friend you have not seen in a long time.

MANAGING THE OPENING MOMENTS OF A CHALLENGING CASE

Every FOP is in the position of having to deal with challenging and sometimes difficult or confrontational patients. In these situations, emotions can easily overtake the content of the conversation, and things can suddenly spiral out of control. An important part of the FOP's job is to help manage these stressful and sometimes awkward situations. When a patient with a problem calls your office or shows up without an appointment to see the hearing care professional, it is important to first recognize which of the three "problem" conditions might apply.

An unhappy customer might arrive at your office in one of three states or conditions: (1) anxious, (2) intimidating, or (3) hostile. The FOP's ability to first recognize the state the patient is in, and then address the condition with the proper communication skills, will help the conversation get off on the right track.

Table 4–5 outlines several typical behaviors related to each of the three conditions. Although not every patient falls into one of these three categories, the majority of hearing-impaired patients will present to your office at one time or another in one of the three states or conditions listed in Table 4–5. Of the three conditions, most hearing-impaired patients will fall into the "Anxious" category, while very few (fortunately) fall into the "Hostile" category.

It is not enough for the FOP to recognize the condition of the customer. Once the condition has been recognized, the FOP must utilize an effective communication strategy in order to find a solution to the problem. One tool that can be used with virtually all customers is called the "Empathy Formula" (Egan, 2007), which is a well-known tool from the field of psychology

Table 4–5. Typical Behaviors to Expect from the Three Conditions of Customers Presenting with a Problem

Anxious	Intimidating	Hostile
Nervous and uncertain	Short, clipped speech	Extremely angry or agitated
Fidgety	Responds with confidence	Points finger to emphasize a point
Indirect eye contact	Direct eye contact	Uses the phrase "you people"
Seems embarrassed	Ready to talk	Sarcastic
May be unwilling to talk about problems	May have a very specific request or problem	Loud voice
Quiet voice		

that gives us the means of keeping the conversation on the right track. There are four steps to the Empathy Formula as shown in Table 4–6.

The Empathy Formula works well for two of the three conditions described in Table 4–5. For the "Anxious" and "Hostile" conditions, the formula is a useful tool for allowing the patient to feel that they have been heard. For example, for a customer arriving at your office with trouble getting the hearing aids into their ears, the Empathy Formula is a useful way to offer reassurance and support, while also allowing the patient a chance to elaborate on the situation causing anxiety and confusion.

On the other hand, the Empathy Formula is not an effective tool for customers presenting in the "Intimidating" condition. For these customers, immediate actions—not words—are required. For example, let us say you have a customer who has visited your office two or three times over the past few months for a minor hearing aid adjustment. The patient, who is getting frustrated, is calling to be seen for a specific hearing aid adjustment, and the FOP tells the patient that it is going to be more than a week before you can fit them into the provider's busy schedule. In this case, using the Empathy Formula might result in upsetting the patient further, turning an "Intimidating" customer into a "Hostile" one. Table 4–7 summarizes some of the actions an FOP can take with difficult or challenging situations, which can occur over the phone or at the front desk.

Once the FOP has successfully booked an appointment, their ability to greet patients, recognize the emotional condition of the patient, and align their communication style to fit the customer's condition cannot be overemphasized. Aside from booking

Table 4–6. The Empathy Formula

Step 1: "You seem . . . "
Step 2: Name the emotion you are observing
Step 3: "about . . . " (Describe the problem or issue causing the emotion)
Step 4: Ask for confirmation and/or clarification ("Is that correct?")

Table 4–7. Suggested Approach for Handling Each of the Three Conditions

Anxious	Intimidating	Hostile
Start with the Empathy Formula	Take immediate action	Start with the Empathy Formula
Use a calm tone of voice	Do not use the Empathy Formula	Isolate them from other patients
Make good eye contact	Stay calm	Encourage them to vent
Emphasize your willingness to help unravel the problem	Attempt to fix the problem with immediate action	Let them know it is acceptable to be angry
Offer reassurance		Try to stay calm
		Offer solutions

an appointment and ensuring that a companion accompany the prospective patient on the first appointment, it is difficult to precisely measure the true financial impact of an effective FOP. Given that an outstanding FOP must reassure a reluctant first-time buyer, calm a nervous patient, or coolly work a frustrated new hearing aid user into a busy schedule, she is an essential part of your sales and marketing team.

Even though they are primarily utilized in the front office for initiating patient contact, the FOP's ability to offer reassurance and support throughout the patient's journey cannot be overemphasized. Considering the strong stigma of hearing aid use, coupled with many of the associated behaviors of untreated sensorineural hearing loss in a predominantly elderly clientele, the job of the FOP is extremely challenging.

Conventional wisdom suggests that a successful hearing aid dispensing practice revolves around the quality of the FOP and

---

@CONNECT

There are many resources available to help boost the skills of FOPs; one can be found at http://www.phonecoach.com/.

his or her ability to provide a remarkable patient experience. Some combination of technical expertise and relationship-building skills is required on the part of the hearing care professional if the office is to be successful.

Although the audiologist's commitment to quality rests with her ability to use best practices in the clinic, perhaps the industry is overlooking the pivotal nature of the unheralded role of the FOP. Taking the time to better hire and train the FOP staff results in a more productive practice with higher levels of quality outcomes for patients.

Here is a simple example of how a commitment to quality affects the overall productivity of a practice. Let us say that you are running a week-long promotional offer in your local newspaper. You are managing two offices that have an average selling price of $2,000 per unit, a close rate of 40%, and a bilateral fitting rate of 80%. In Office 1, the FOP is poorly trained, whereas in Office 2, you have taken the time to hire the right person and invested the necessary time to train this person on the essential job duties. In this example, let us also say that you received on average 12 calls per day over a 1-week period in each office inquiring about the promotion. Table 4–2 shows the difference between the revenue generated when all the other key operational variables stayed the same between the two offices. It is a good example of how better quality improves overall productivity.

#DISCOVER

The Quality Equation

Behavior = Performance = Results

If you are trying to improve the outcome of something, you need to start by identifying the behaviors that are most likely to contribute to optimal results or outcomes. The Pareto rule suggests that 20% of the FOP's daily activities contributes to 80% of their productivity. The critical 20% is likely related to many of the FOP's behaviors as outlined in this chapter.

REFERENCES

Egan, G. (2007). *Exercises in helping skills* (8th ed.). Pacific Grove, CA: Pacific Grove Books.

Mehrabian, A., & Wiener, M. (1967). Decoding of inconsistent communications. *Journal of Personality and Social Psychology, 6*(1), 109–114.

5

QUALITY IN THE BUSINESS SUITE

In a book devoted to quality let us begin the final chapter by examining what many think of as its analogue, productivity. Although quality is mainly related to *how well* something gets done, productivity pertains to *what* or *how often* something gets done. Conventional wisdom suggests that in a low-volume, high-margin medically oriented business, such as hearing aid dispensing, the three key drivers of productivity are office traffic, units sold, and average selling price. If you can manage these three key variables by infusing them with many of the quality principles put forth in this book, your practice is likely to experience consistent, double-digit, year-over-year revenue growth.

This chapter reviews several essential business management principles as they relate to quality. The material is mainly geared toward clinicians who find themselves thrust into the role of practice manager. Let us look at each of these three drivers of productivity, which are shown in Figure 5–1, more closely. Office traffic is the number of patients seeking your services and is mainly a function of marketing and reputation. Of course, if your reputation is based on high-quality service delivery, it is likely

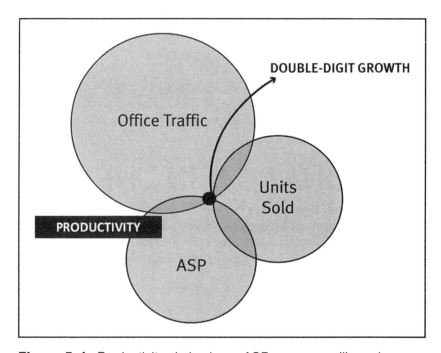

Figure 5–1. Productivity circles here. *ASP,* average selling price.

that you will reap the rewards of high levels of office traffic generated from word-of-mouth referrals. (Word-of-mouth referrals are considered the gold standard by which a practice generates additional traffic because the return on investment is essentially zero.) The second key driver of productivity is the number of hearing aids (often referred to as units) sold. The number of units sold is typically measured by looking at the number of opportunities (an opportunity is defined as an individual presenting in your practice with an "aidable" hearing loss, motivated to try hearing aids) that actually make a decision to purchase hearing aids at the end of the appointment. Units sold is usually measured and tracked with a ratio called the close rate. Close rate is the number of patients who agree to purchase hearing aids on the day of their consultation appointment divided by the number of opportunities. Another common way to evaluate units sold is to track the binaural rate of your practice.

The third key driver of productivity in a hearing aid dispensing practice is average selling price (ASP). For every device that is sold, it is imperative that its retail price be tracked. Retail price, of course, is what the patient (or insurance company) paid for the hearing aids. A slightly different way to gauge ASP is through product mix. Product mix is typically evaluated by tracking how many devices are dispensed along three or four technology tiers. For the novice manager having a maniacal focus on these three productivity variables, it is a great starting point for creating a profitable practice.

Quality in the business suite is largely based on the manager's ability to wrap processes and metrics around these three key drivers of productivity. As you may have guessed after reading the first four chapters of this book, standardization of processes (behaviors) and benchmarking are the heart of productivity. Before delving into the details of benchmarking and the use of key performance indicators (KPIs), let us look at what managers need to get right in order to ensure that their business is both profitable and highly reputable.

BUILDING A PRACTICE BASED ON TEAMWORK AND INTEGRITY

Imagine you have bought a practice that has been in existence for 25 years. Your due diligence told you that even though the practice was profitable, it suffered from a less than stellar reputation in your community. As you take a leap of faith into the world of private practice or management of one owned by someone else, you are concerned that the legacy of this business will limit your ability to grow it. What quality principles can you apply that will not only improve the reputation of the business, but allow its revenue to grow? This next section will provide guidance on this all too common scenario.

Using several of the quality principles discussed in previous chapters, let us explore how to apply them in the management of a private practice. (Even if you do not own a private practice, these principles still apply if you are employed in a medical center, hospital, hearing aid shop, or any other dispensing business in which you are making decisions.) Before you have hung your shingle with your name on the outside of your door stating to the world you are open for business, the first task is to clearly define what you want your business to represent. More than a mission statement, this requires that you take the time to think through your values and how they apply to the running of your practice. Values can be defined as broad preferences concerning appropriate courses of action or outcome. Values reflect a person's sense of right and wrong or what "ought" to be. "Equal rights for all," "Excellence deserves admiration," and "People should be treated with respect and dignity" are representative of personal values. Values tend to influence attitudes and behavior, and because of these reasons they form the foundation for how you want to manage your practice. Another word for values is "ethics." You can think of values or ethics as what you are willing to do—even when no one is looking. In practical terms, values (or ethics) deal with the "right" conduct and "leading a good life." Are you in the business primarily to extract wealth over a short period of time or do you desire to be a long-standing member of your local business community? An honest answer to this question helps to define your values. When asked this important question, just about everyone would answer that they are in business to serve people and be an upstanding member of the community, but what counts are your actions. Perhaps a better question, therefore, is do your actions exemplify short-term extractive business practices or community-based, inclusive principles? It is a critical question to ponder because your core values determine the direction of the business. Only after you have deliberately thought through your personal values, and how they can be applied to the management of your practice, can you begin the processing of building a practice known for high quality.

Business leaders are by law accountable to their shareholders for their Profit and Loss statements. Due to the Sarbanes-Oxley Act, CEOs can go to jail when they mislead the public about their company's financial performance. On the other hand, owners of smaller health care organizations, such as hearing aid dispensing practices, are largely immune to regulations that govern issues that concern core values; thus, it requires owners and managers of audiology practices to govern their own behaviors and actions by relying on their own core values. Among the core values that assist private practice owners in running an ethical business devoted to high-quality patient care are integrity and teamwork.

There, of course, are several core values upon which one could build their practice. Hard work, ethical practice, and entrepreneurial spirit are just a few that come to mind. It is really up to the individual practice owner or manager to decide which core values have the highest priority and need to be woven into the practice's culture. The examples we use are the core values of integrity and teamwork. Put most simply, integrity is having the courage to follow one's convictions. Stephen Carter, author and professor, defines integrity as a process that entails the following: (1) One must take pains to try to discern what is right or wrong; (2) One must be willing to shape one's actions in accord with that discernment, even when it is difficult or painful to do so; and (3) One must be willing to acknowledge publicly what one is doing. In short, a person of integrity must be reflective, steadfast, trustworthy, and *whole*. As Carter (1997) states, "A person of integrity . . . is a whole person, a person somehow undivided." Carter's process-oriented definition of integrity fits well with quality practice management, as it takes into consideration doing the right thing with respect to patient care and allowing the results of it to be transparent—even when no one is looking.

@*CONNECT*

Dave Logan and Core Values

Dave Logan and Tribal Leadership have designed a unique package of coaching tools to make you a better leader, upgrade the culture of your organization, and dramatically improve the results of your business. Dave can be followed on Twitter @culturesync.

Teamwork, on the other hand, is a core value that represents collective action and the thoughtful division of labor within a practice. Mayo Clinic, which has teamwork as a core value, is known for outstanding levels of quality. For audiologists, Mayo Clinic represents a good example of a culture devoted to teamwork.

Practice owners and managers would be wise to adapt many of their strategies that foster teamwork. When the core value of teamwork is infused throughout the organization everyone is working toward the same goal of reducing variability in outcome and providing comprehensive care. Devising specific actions through a documented best practice protocol along six patient interaction stations, such as the one outlined in Chapter 1, is an example of putting the core value of teamwork into action. Each staff member is accountable for completing a set of specific tasks as they relate to patient care. Additionally, the core value of teamwork necessitates the use of metrics that evaluate how effective your team is performing. For example, a survey question could ask patients to judge the effectiveness of your team on a 1–5 Likert scale.

The process of building a practice on a sound foundation of integrity and teamwork revolves around three components: people, process, and tools. They are sometimes known as the management trinity as shown in Figure 5–2. When these three components are working harmoniously, the end result is likely

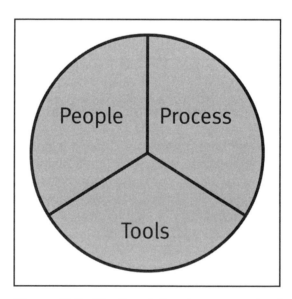

Figure 5–2. The foundational components of any organization. Also known as "the management trinity."

to be a profitable business that is known for delivering high-quality outcomes.

Although it is a cliché, the people that you hire form the foundation for the results and reputation of your practice. Since we discussed hiring processes in Chapter 4, we do not go into the details here, except to say that the staff you hire for your practice must represent your core values. The next pillar that your practice rests on is process. Process can be defined as the way in which your business operates. In addition to the clinical processes you conduct, there are several other business management processes that need to be thought through and implemented. Some examples include what key performance metrics of your practice you will measure, how often you will evaluate these metrics, and how you will create actions around gaps in performance relative to benchmarks. The final components of the foundational pillars are tools. Tools represent the tactics and skills your team needs to get the job done. Anything from diagnostic equipment to computers to training represent things that are needed to generate positive results and optimize patient care.

@CONNECT

GE People Matrix: "Broom 'em or Groom 'em"

In large, highly competitive organizations, finding the right people to fill key roles within the organization is paramount to long-term success. General Electric has pioneered the use of a "people matrix" that allows managers to rate both the performance of the individual and their core values. Using a 1 to 10 scale (10 is an unattainably perfect score) managers can rate both the performance and the values of each employee. Individuals that rank highly on both scales are top priority for career development and advancement within the organization. Both low performers and those that rank below par on the core value scale are candidates to be weeded out of the organization. The former CEO of GE, Jack Welch, pioneered this concept. He can be followed on Twitter at @jack_welch.

The wide-scale use of training and coaching in order to implement best practices and behaviorally based standards are examples of tools. In summary, effective managers find people that match their core values, create processes that maximize their efficiency, and identify tools that are needed to optimize results.

Once an overarching strategy (either to grow or maintain your current business) has been developed, it is crucial that the manager or owner create some specific strategic imperatives. Strategic imperatives is another term for priorities. Some examples of universal strategic imperatives that any business may wish to prioritize include operational excellence, patient experience, and teamwork. Another way to think about strategic imperatives is that they are potential competitive advantages. This means that your business has achieved such an outstanding level of performance in a certain area that it becomes a defining reason for your success. There are many examples of companies that outperform their competitors because they offer customers something that the competition cannot offer. Walmart, for example, has a strong competitive advantage around inventory management and logistics. Through their use of data, they know precisely how many of a certain item is needed on each shelf. Through this competitive advantage they can pass on a lower retail price compared with their competitors. Audiologists and hearing instrument professionals do not have competitive advantages surrounding inventory, logistics, and supply-chain management, but they can develop strong competitive advantages around other things. Operational excellence is the practice's ability to control costs, optimize profitability, and, generally, run an efficient organization. If a practice can see patients faster (without a 3-week wait time), move them through the appointment cycles efficiently (fewer returns for credit and optimal patient satisfaction in less than a month), or use their buying power to lower their cost of goods, the practice is using operational excellence as a competitive advantage.

Another possible competitive advantage is providing a memorable patient experience. If you offer an interaction with patients that is so remarkable and rooted in creating a strong transformational bond between patient and provider, this can become a competitive advantage. Several "helping" professions, such as medicine, teaching, and nursing, are naturally inclined toward building competitive advantages around the patient experience.

Strategic imperatives that become competitive advantages not only allow a practice to differentiate itself from competitors, but they also represent value in the eyes of entrepreneurs who may desire to acquire your practice. In other words, your competitive advantage is an asset that others may be interested in acquiring.

Once you have a handle on your strategic imperatives, it is critical that you develop strategic tactics to support them. Specific procedures or behaviors, such as many outlined in Chapters 3 and 4, represent strategic tactics. For each strategic initiative it is critical to create three to five specific strategic tactics that can be put in place by your staff. For example, the strategic tactics executed by front office professionals are found in Chapter 4, while many of the strategic tactics executed by clinicians are found in Chapter 3. For the business manager who is accountable for cost control, top-line growth, and bottom-line profit, day-to-day activities related to each must be in alignment with the core values of the business. An example of these tactics with respect to retail pricing is covered later in this chapter.

#DISCOVER

Strategy Versus Tactic

You have probably noticed the word "strategic" used in a couple of different ways. The two most critical terms are "strategy" and "tactic." A strategy is *how* you plan to bring your services to market or grow your business. For example, building a business that attempts to capture the premium segment of the market is a strategy. A tactic, on the other hand, is what you are planning to do in order to fulfill your strategy. Creating a memorable clinical experience for patients along six distinct interaction stations would be an example of a group of specific tactics. A clear strategy with specific tactics to support it is a key to effective, quality management.

GOALS AND OBJECTIVES FOR STAFF

Once the strategic tactics of a business have been created and each member of the staff has a solid understanding of how their day-to-day tasks affect them, the manager can devise goals and objectives for each staff member. Goals and objectives are a list of no more than two to three actionable tasks that are expected to be completed by each member of the staff. Much has been written in various business management texts and articles about how to write goals. The main point stressed here is that from a quality management perspective goals and objectives are instrumental in ensuring the practice is standardizing self-improvement and productivity. In other words, managers work with each member of the staff to identify their key role within the business for improving quality of care or overall productivity. For example, an audiologist might have the goal of adding one new hearing aid consultation per day to their schedule. This would serve as the goal. Objectives would be the step-by-step process the audiologist and manager have created to attain this goal. Once the goals and objectives have been created, the audiologist and manager meet on a monthly basis to review key performance indicators (KPIs) that help determine if progress toward the goal is being made and what modifications or help is needed to get on track. KPIs are the data that are needed to make decisions about progress toward a goal and need to be reviewed at least on a monthly basis.

@CONNECT

Peter Drucker

A pioneer in the field of business management, Peter Drucker authored dozens of books and articles over a career that spanned five decades. One of his most famous quotes is, "Effective management is to have one or two clear priorities; having more than two is a circus." Learn more by following the Drucker Institute on Twitter @DruckerInst.

KEY PERFORMANCE INDICATORS

Key performance indicators (KPIs) are the navigation instruments used by managers to understand their business and whether it is on a successful track or needs to change course. Like a captain relies on his instruments to pilot the ship, the manager relies on his own KPI dashboard to steer her business. There are dozens of KPIs that can be tracked on a daily, weekly, monthly, or annual basis. The challenge for any manager is to find the right set of KPIs to monitor over time. Many managers fall into the trap of trying to measure too many things and get lost in a sea of data. This section attempts to provide the manager with a reasonable number of KPIs to evaluate on a routine basis in order to navigate the overall productivity and quality of the practice.

Key performance indicators are used in all walks of life. For example, dieters use calorie-counting apps on their iPhone and a scale to manage weight loss. Baseball managers evaluate pitch count and earned run average, among other key stats, to monitor the performance of their pitching staff. In these examples, notice there are both leading and lagging KPIs. A combination of leading and lagging KPIs are critical to managing a pitching staff, your health, and a business. In the case of the baseball manager, the pitch count is one leading KPI of results, as the higher the pitch count, the more likely it is for the pitcher to tire and perform poorly. For the dieter, caloric count is a lead indicator of weight loss, as lower calorie consumption leads to weight loss.

In an audiology practice, a lead KPI is telling you something about performance or results *before* revenue has been generated or a patient has been fitted with hearing aids; thus, it is a lead KPI. It is important to focus on one or two lead KPIs since they provide important red flags about what is happening in the process of generating revenue or serving a patient. On the other hand, a lagging KPI tells you something that has already happened. Similar to the baseball box score, a lagging KPI provides you with information that you cannot act upon, at least in the short term. The key point is that you need to look at one or two leading and lagging KPIs on a routine basis. Lagging KPIs are like reading the box score of your favorite baseball team in the newspaper the morning after Saturday night's game. It gives you a lot of interesting information, but there is no action you can take to change the outcome of the game. On the other hand, leading indicators provide data-driven insight into results before they occur; therefore, you can take immediate action to change an outcome. The bottom line is that lead KPIs are an absolutely necessary part of managing for quality. A good example of a leading KPI is appointments made and number of patients evaluated. If these numbers are low, then you need to do something quickly to improve the final result. Conversely, lagging KPIs include net profit, revenue, and number of units sold. These are facts that tell you a lot about the business, but they capture information about the past; thus, it is nearly impossible to take immediate action when these lagging KPIs are lower than expected. You can act upon the information, but it takes a lot longer to turn these numbers around because they are telling you something about past behavior and performance.

Two KPI terms that one hears quite often are dashboard and scorecard.

You can think of both as tools that summarize leading and lagging KPIs of your business. Once you have evaluated the data in the form of a dashboard or scorecard, you can make decisions about your business and take action based on the numbers you see. Below are some examples of KPI dashboards that are needed to effectively manage the quality and productivity of a business, along with some insights on how to create your own.

Productivity Dashboard

You can devise your own productivity dashboard by asking yourself, "What are the essential activities that generate revenue in my practice?" The answer to that question is likely to provide you with the three KPIs that need to be tracked on a daily or weekly basis. Also, included is some benchmark data from a recently published survey (Phonak, 2012). (From Chapter 2 you should know that benchmarks serve as a method of comparing performance with some well-defined, data-driven standards.) These KPIs are as follows:

- Number of appointments per week. This is a lead KPI that tells you how many opportunities you have to generate revenue. Since each patient represents an opportunity to deliver service, you can track number of appointments as a lead indicator. Survey data suggest that the average office with one full-time clinician sees approximately 30 to 40 opportunities per month. This serves as a benchmark.

- Unit sales by office/provider per month. This is arguably a lead, rather than a lagging KPI. Since the patient is likely to agree to the purchase without paying for it completely, we consider it a leading KPI. (You cannot count the sale as money in the bank until the return privilege is over.) Survey data suggest that the average practice dispensers between 17 and 20 units per month in a single-provider practice. This figure serves as a reasonable benchmark for the practice with a single practitioner that is open all day, five days per week, which is considered a full-time office.

- Gross margin for each device dispensed, tracked by clinician per month. A lagging KPI of productivity is gross margin per clinician. Gross margin is the difference between the retail price and cost of goods sold per device, expressed as a dollar value. According to survey data, the median gross margin in the United States is 55% per device dispensed. This means that 45% of the retail cost of each hearing aid is paid to the manufacturer. The figure of 55% gross margin per instrument serves as a benchmark relative to industry norms. As a best practice, Brady (2010) recommends a gross margin per device of approximately 60 to 65%.

There are dozens of other productivity KPIs that can be tracked, including close rate, product mix, and binaural rate. The important points are that each practice needs to identify two to three KPIs to track on a weekly or monthly basis. The three KPIs listed above, which are composed of two leading indicators, and one lagging indicator, of productivity, are usually the most critical to monitor weekly and monthly. Even though benchmarks were also included for these three measures, practices are strongly advised to create their own benchmarks after carefully evaluating their breakeven expenses and other costs of running their practice.

There, of course, are a few other KPIs that need to be evaluated on a monthly or semiannual basis. Revenue and profit statements should be evaluated on a monthly basis. Since these are lagging indicators of a business, they are not immediately actionable. Nevertheless, they provide critical information about the overall health of the business. As a benchmark, practices should obtain a pretax profit margin of 10% (Crabtree, 2011). A final word on productivity metrics is warranted. Notice in Figure 5–3 that KPIs are tracked using a line graph. Line graphs provide a quick visual snapshot of performance over several months. Line graphs like the ones shown in Figure 5–3 allow you to make a quick comparison between providers or locations. Moreover, even though they are not shown in Figure 5–3, benchmarks can be added on a line graph, usually in the form of a horizontal red line; thus, managers can quickly see how far below (or above) performance is relative to the benchmark. Most computerized office management systems allow you to develop reports in line-graph form. Excel spreadsheets can also easily be converted to line graphs.

Quality Scorecard

Another set of KPIs that must be tracked on a weekly or monthly basis are devoted to quality of care delivered to patients. These are generally considered leading KPIs because you can act upon the information before revenue is generated. Like productivity KPIs, each quality KPI needs to have a data-driven benchmark. There are dozens of quality KPIs that can be tracked, such as defect rate of products received from the manufacturer and repair rates. The two quality KPIs listed below probably have the most practical value; therefore, they are provided in more detail:

- Returns for credit. In simple terms, returns for credit are the dollar value of all products that are exchanged or refunded. Notice that in this definition we are using dollars, not units, as the critical variable. When a simple calculation of returns is used, rather than dollars, some information critical to quality is not captured.

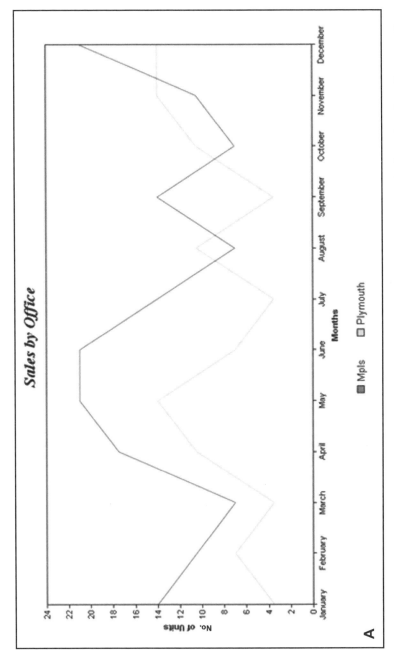

Figure 5–3. A–C. Example of line-graph reports for unit sales and gross margin for a two-location practice. (Courtesy of Bill Savage, AudServ, Inc.) *(continues)*

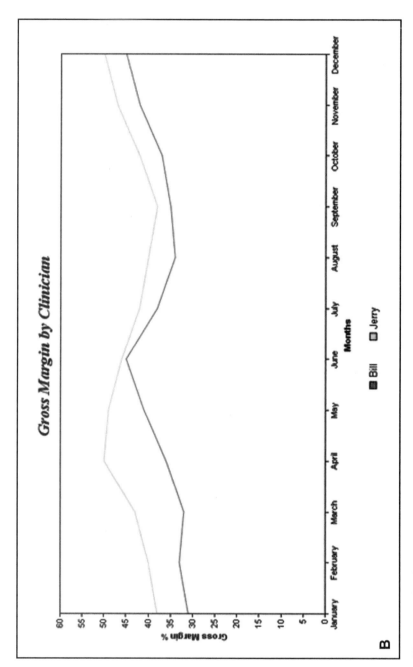

Figure 5–3. *(continues)*

236

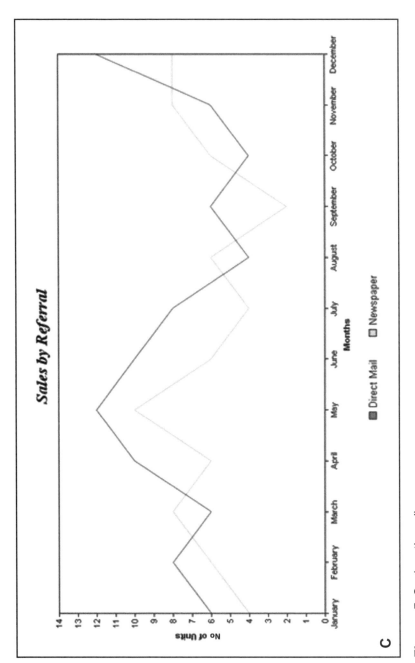

Figure 5-3. *(continued)*

237

For example, let us say that you have a practice that is doing a lot of exchanging of premium products for economy-level products. Technically, there is an exceptionally low return rate since all of the patients end up wearing the device, albeit low-end products, after an arduous trial process with premium products first. By using dollars, rather than units, to track returns and exchanges, this gap in the practice—exchanging premium for economy—is quickly uncovered. As a basic rule of thumb, no more than 7 to 10% of total revenue should be refunded back to patients in the form of a return or exchange.

■ Patient satisfaction/benefit. Another quality KPI that received our attention in Chapter 3 is patient benefit and satisfaction. (Patient satisfaction surveys and outcome measures are reviewed extensively there.) Both patient benefit and satisfaction can be tracked as a quality KPI using a scorecard, such as the one shown in Figure 5–4.

Quality Scorecard

Patient Name: _____

Audiologist: _____

Date of fit: _____

Date of final evaluation: _____

12-point check	Comments:
o Hearing evaluated in sound-proof booth	_____
o Speech-in-noise tests completed	_____
o Results and recommendations explained in detail	_____
o Hearing aid features explained in detail	_____
o Orientation to devices	_____
o REM/objective performance measures	_____
o Physical fit is acceptable (1 = poor, 5 = outstanding)	_____
o Sound quality is acceptable (1 = poor, 5 = outstanding)	_____
o Performance in background noise (1 = poor, 5 = outstanding)	_____
o Average usage time per day	_____ hours per day
o Aided TELEGRAM	_____
o Overall real-world benefit (1 = poor, 5 = outstanding)	_____

_____ Patient Signature   _____ Audiologist Signature

Figure 5–4. Example of a quality scorecard or checklist.

This scorecard can be completed by the patient several weeks after their fitting, perhaps at a 3-month checkup. Patients can complete this scorecard independently or with some assistance from the service provider. The scorecard could also be mailed to patients a month or two after the fitting. Scores can be compiled, which then serve as benchmark data for the practice.

In addition to quality and productivity KPIs, practices would be wise to use financial and marketing KPIs. Examples of financial KPIs include net profit, net profit margin, and EBITDA. Although

---

#DISCOVER

The Book *Moneyball* by Michael Lewis

Moneyball can teach managers the following five lessons about data-driven decision making:

1. Always focus on the results you want to achieve regardless of your budget and current position. Low budget does not always mean you cannot compete against the top players in your industry.
2. Measure the right things. Avoid bias, old habits, and the way business has been done for years. Focus on different priorities and what really drives your business results.
3. Be willing to take risks based on your numbers. If you measure the right things and you understand your numbers, you can build a winning strategy. Act on your information and take the risk.
4. Give the support and training to your team to succeed. Different strategies require different team-building approaches to achieve the highest performance.
5. Discipline in implementation. Believe in your strategy, live your strategy, and stick to it. If you have done your homework and made decisions based on relevant facts, stick to your strategy and continuously improve your team performance, and the results will come.

these KPIs are well beyond the scope of a book devoted to quality, you can consult your accountant or other trusted financial advisor; however, they are at least worth mentioning here. Additionally, since marketing is critical to productivity and growth of a practice, having one or two marketing KPIs is warranted. Cost per lead and conversion rate are a couple of marketing KPIs that you can track.

MANAGEMENT DECISIONS IN THE HIRING PROCESS

Knowing when to hire another person for your practice is one of the most critical decisions an owner or manager will ever make. This is largely because the price of labor is high and relatively fixed. According to Crabtree (2011) the pretax profit of a business needs to be at least 10% of total annual revenue before hiring another person for your staff. (If you did not generate a 10% pretax profit in the previous year, you probably need to hold your labor cost constant.) If your pretax profit is 10% or more of your total revenue, then you can begin the process of hiring another person for your staff. The two major reasons for bringing another person on board is generating more revenue (and profit) and/or lessening your own workload. The former represents a challenge surrounding the division of labor, while the latter signifies a change in your role within the organization akin to shareholder, rather than audiologist/owner. Regardless of the specific reason, it is important that you carefully evaluate the efficiency of your labor.

Once you know you can afford to hire another person, you need to carefully decide how this new staff member will contribute to the profitability of your business. In general, there are three ways to divide your labor force:

■ Staff that bring more patients to your practice through marketing. These are the "finders" within your practice.
■ Staff that take care of the patients through consultative selling and clinical efforts. These are the "minders" in your practice.

■ Staff that take care of the essential back office activities, such as phone scheduling, billing, and coding. These are the "grinders" in your practice.

Of course, in many practices the same person plays all three roles simultaneously. Also, there certainly are times when you may want to contract an outside agency or consultant for special projects or assignments. If you are the owner or manager of your practice, some of the practical questions you need to ask yourself before adding to your head count include:

■ Will you have more time to market your services and expand your business?
■ Will bringing a new person on board allow you to dispense more products or serve more patients?
■ Will you be able to give your patients more efficient service or quicker delivery, with the result that higher quality would lead to additional patients?

Unfortunately, there are few resources that offer guidance on when to hire and how to divide labor within a practice in order to improve productivity. The purpose of this section is to offer some practical insight and guidance as they relate to the management of quality.

Believe it or not, running a profitable audiology or hearing aid dispensing practice has more in common with the National Football League (NFL) than you might think. For about the past 20 years the NFL has operated under a salary cap. The main objective of the salary cap is to control the costs of labor and ensure parity by requiring that all teams spend the same amount of money on its labor force, which are the players. In 2012 each NFL team had about $120 million to spend on a roster of 53 players. If each player on the 53-man roster was paid equally, each would receive about $2.3 million per year. Of course, each player does not receive equal pay, as some positions and players are considered to be much more valuable; thus, a considerably higher salary is warranted.

As previously mentioned, a salary cap enables teams to control costs. This helps prevent situations in which a club signs a high-cost player in order to reap the rewards of success immediately, only to later find themselves in financial difficulty because of those high costs as the player's skills diminish over time. Without caps there is a risk that teams will overspend in order to win now at the expense of long-term stability. Salary caps incentivize teams to develop talent over time. This is more likely to lead to team stability, which is important for fans. No one wants to see their team lose year after year, or worse yet, go completely out of business.

Like most other professionals sports, a salary cap is something that is mandated by the NFL commissioner. Teams cannot choose not to follow it. For teams that exceed the salary cap, there are severe penalties that could jeopardize the competitiveness of the team in future years. Private businesses, on the other hand, do not have the luxury of following a mandated salary to keep their labor costs in check. Even though they are not required to hold their costs in line with a salary cap, using "salary-cap thinking" is an effective way to know when you can bring a new employee into the business and at what approximate pay grade.

What Is Your Salary Cap?

As a general statement, labor productivity is what powers sustainable businesses. This means that business owners must find the proper balance between what tasks the staff perform during the work day and at what dollar amount the staff is paid to perform those tasks. In other words, you and your staff have to be busy, but you have to be busy doing the things that lead to optimizing revenue for your business over the course of a day, month, or year.

Regardless of how you specifically measure labor efficiency in your office, the idea of a salary cap is a great way to achieve business goals without overspending on the costs of labor. Let us work through a simple example of how an audiology practice owner might determine their salary cap using a couple of assumptions. Most experts suggest that a business needs at least 10% pretax profit to be sustainable. This pretax profit is not used to pay salaries, but is set aside to reinvest in the infrastructure of the business or to cover expenses for a particularly poor month of low sales or high returns. In addition, we know that the combination of hearing aid cost of goods and other expenses, such as marketing, rent, and utilities need to be around 50% of gross revenue. These assumptions are shown in Table 5–1 for a practice that has been in existence for more than 10 years. (The $1 million mark was chosen because it is a nice round number, not because it represents any type of benchmark!) In this example, the owner, who happens to be an AuD-trained audiologist, has toiled for more than a decade building this practice from scratch and is faced with the knotty decision of whether or not to hire a recent AuD graduate from the local university, an experienced clinical audiologist with sales experience, another assistant, or not hire anyone at this time.

By accounting for a pretax profit of 10% and all direct costs (excluding labor), we are able to get a clear idea of how much we can afford for labor *before* we make any hiring decision. In Table 5–1, for example, the salary cap is $400,000, which represents 40% of the total annual revenue of that practice. This is the amount of money the practice has to spend on labor, including the salary of the audiologist/owner. In an ideal world, you might be tempted to bring on one or two more "star performers" (e.g., experienced, doctorate-level audiologist) to maintain this half-million dollars in gross profit, along with the expectation that the business will experience double-digit growth over time. The reality, however, is much different since each of those proven

Table 5–1. Financials from a Private Practice

Revenue	$1,000,000
Direct costs (excludes labor), for example, cost of goods, marketing, rent, utilities (50%)	($500,000)
Gross profit	$500,000
Salary cap (40%)	($400,000)
Total expenses	($900,000)
Pretax profit (10%)	$100,000

star performers are likely to command a premium salary of about $150,000 annually, plus benefits. (If you add the usual 33% of the salary for benefits, that brings that salary to $199,500 per star.) The math in Table 5–1 dictates that we have to be extremely cautious is our hiring decisions.

Let us take a more careful look at the salary cap of this practice, which employs one audiologist/owner and two full-time assistants who are responsible for billing, coding, marketing, and answering the phone, among other necessary activities. Table 5–2 provides a breakdown of labor expenses relative to the salary cap.

The available cap space tells us that this practice has $66,500 to spend on another staff member. Using the salary cap as the primary guide in making the decision to hire another professional, we realize there is a rather stark choice between three possibilities:

1. The first-round draft choice. Hire that new AuD graduate who is a potential star performer at well below the market value. Under this scenario, the star performer would accept a salary plus benefits of $66,500 with the expectation of growing the business over a finite period of time. This choice may be most appropriate if the audiologist/owner wants to continue with her current work load while continuing to grow the practice and eventually transition out of the business.
2. The proven free agent with a high-performance track record. Hire an existing star performer at current market value.

Table 5–2. Labor Costs for a Private Practice

	Salary + Benefits
Audiologist/owner	$199,500
Assistant 1	$77,000
Assistant 2	$57,000
Total	$333,500
Cap space	$66,500

Under this scenario, the proven star performer would command compensation of roughly $200,000 (salary plus benefits). Since this is well over the salary cap, the audiologist/owner could choose to stop actively seeing patients or drop to part-time status and receive a dividend from pretax profits rather than a high salary plus benefits.

3. The free-agent "utility man" (a baseball term that refers to a player who can play more than one position). The third choice would be for the audiologist/owner to continue with their current workload and bring another assistant into the fold that could conduct some of the testing, follow-up with repairs, as well as other front office and back office duties. This person could be an audiology assistant who may be eligible to obtain a state license to dispense hearing aids.

Now the numbers can be worked backward to see how much labor is going to be needed to service those patients that generated $500,000 in annual gross profit. In order to know which hiring choice is best for you, let us look at some other data from this practice in Table 5–3.

The real question is how many workers do you need to service 100 new patients and 220 experienced patients that repurchased products, in addition to taking care of hundreds more of existing patients you are likely to see over the course of the year. Let us assume that it takes an average of 4.5 hours of time for 1 year to service new patients, and an average of 3 hours of

Table 5–3. Key Variables for a Private Practice

Revenue from the sale of hearing aids	$850,000
Revenue from testing, service contracts, batteries, etc.	$150,000
Total number of patients in database	4,000
Total number of patients who purchased last year	220
New patients who purchased last year	100
Total units dispensed last year	380

time to service an experienced patient fitted with new hearing aids. For the 220 patients fitted with hearing aids, that amounts to 690 cumulative hours of the audiologist/owner's time. Let us compare these numbers to the capacity of each professional in your practice.

Division of Labor

The key to staying under your salary cap is the judicious use of support personnel. After all, it is oftentimes the middling utility player that bales the star out of an ineffective performance by delivering a hit in crunch time! With a salary cap, your practice must rely on the utility player to deliver in the clutch.

Support personnel within the practice (the free-agent utility player) must accept the role of jack-of-all-trades within the organization. In addition to conducting the essential work scheduling appointments, other duties may include hearing aid cleaning and troubleshooting, conducting hearing aid orientation classes, and facilitating physician marketing campaigns. (Please check with your state licensing board to see what licenses and credentials are needed to complete some of these tasks.) According to our calculations, each support staff has 1,840 hr available for the year to contribute to generating revenue by serving patients in various capacities.

Let us turn our attention to the daily workload of the star performer. You might be wondering, "What is the maximum volume that the star performer can handle, or even should handle, before work quality starts deteriorating?" The answer to that question is not an easy one because it depends on the staff member; however, after almost 30 years of working with many different audiologists with various years of experience, it has been our observation that audiologists can suffer burnout if scheduled for more than 7 hr of direct patient contact per day during a 5-day work week. In a typical setting, after vacations, sick time, and "administration" time are taken into consideration, the audiologist has about 1,380 hr of clinical time per year to see patients (6 hr per business day).

In this scenario the audiologist/owner is using 50% of their clinical time to fit patients (1,380 total clinical hours/690 hr). Since the audiologist/owner still has about half of her time available to see existing patients for annual follow-ups, hearing screenings, and so forth, it probably does not make sense to hire another star performer unless the current audiologist/owner wants to transition to shareholder status. Fortunately, this practice has two ambitious support staff that can play the role of utility players by providing a range of services for the practice; therefore, this audiologist needs to be efficient with her time, rather than hire another star performer—even if that star decides to work for less than their market value. Assuming the audiologist/owner wants to continue to see patients on a full-time basis, the decision to bring in a first-round draft choice or star free agent should be delayed until she is at 80% or more of full capacity seeing new and existing patients for hearing aid fittings.

Support personnel are being used successfully in a variety of practice settings, including the military, the Veterans Administration, educational institutions, hospitals, industrial settings, and private practices. History has shown that the use of support personnel can be a tremendous asset to an audiology practice, both by improving productivity and by increasing profitability and patient satisfaction. It would seem that delegating tasks that do not require the educational and expertise of a hearing professional to support personnel would allow the professionals to see more patients, potentially generating more revenue which could lead to increased profitability. Just imagine how many more patients you could see if you did not have to clean hearing aids, complete order and repair forms, set up testing procedures, troubleshoot equipment, teach patients how to clean, insert, and remove hearing aids, not to mention demonstrating how to use remote controls, t-coils, auditory trainingprograms, loop systems, and other assistive devices. You could actually spend more time providing vitally needed services such as family counseling, outlining realistic expectations, performing speech-in-noise testing, assessing central processing function, and developing relationships with your patients as well as referring physicians.

The decision to hire another staff member is never a capricious one. Regardless of the status of the employee you are targeting to bring on-board, that is, star free agent, first-round draft pick, or utility man, both a salary cap and calculation of labor efficiency can be used to make a data-driven decision. Of course, the supply and demand of your local labor market coupled with the overall pretax profitability of your practice contribute to your hiring decision. As a general rule, however, practitioners should work to maximize the overall productivity of their existing staff before hiring another person.

Managing Quality in the Age of Transparency

Here is a story to illustrate the importance of quality in changing times: I was driving through my neighborhood the other day and noticed that several cameras had been installed on the traffic lights near busy intersections. In addition to the new cameras, two new speed limit signs were equipped with flashing lights that are triggered when approaching vehicles exceed the 35 mph speed limit.

There is nothing terribly ominous about the presence of cameras in all sorts of places these days. Studies even show that their mere presence on the roadways significantly reduces accidents. About the same time those traffic cameras were installed, I discovered that hospitals are beginning to use cameras to record surgical procedures.

Now, like NFL players and coaches, surgical teams are able to review their performance and critique it shortly thereafter. Some physicians even provide their patient with a link to their videotaped procedure, so that it can be kept in the patient's electronic medical records. When you consider the relatively high error rate of surgery, greater transparency in health care is definitely a good thing most of the time.

Greater transparency also has a down side. We live in an age when virtually all aspects of our personal lives are accessible to anyone with a laptop computer, wireless Internet connection, and basic hacking skills. The reality is that information about you and your practice can no longer be kept private.

A simple Google search of your practice is likely to yield patient ratings on a myriad of sites such as Yelp and Health-Grades.com. Even Facebook is beginning to offer reviews and grades of professional service firms by qualified individuals. Of course, our practices have always been at the mercy of over-zealous or disgruntled individuals who, for no good reason, may spread negative information to their relatively small circle of friends and acquaintances. Today, however, online tools allow millions of people to read such reviews—no matter how unfounded or scurrilous they may be.

The age of transparency is the result of the convergence of two forces that are likely to be with us for years to come. The first force is something information technology experts call "Big Data," which is the collection, analysis, storage, synthesis, and sharing of digital information.

Much as hearing aid algorithms can recognize the listening environment of the individual and automatically shift processing strategies to optimize speech intelligibility, sophisticated algorithms can recognize your buying preferences and instantaneously shift the advertising you see to conform to your tastes and desires. It is scary to realize that your opinions, preferences, habits, and history can be gathered almost instantly and boiled down to an algorithm. For the owner or manager of a business, the presence of Big Data may be so overwhelming that you do not know what to do with all of it.

The second prevailing force is a strong desire by many people to network, opine, and rant from the virtual, remote comforts of their laptop, tablet computer, or smartphone. Some refer to this as the "Facebook Effect." In the virtual word of Twitter and other social media in which you are not engaged in direct face-to-face communication, it is easy to say outlandish and downright strange things.

In an age of transparency, where your every move can be tracked, discussed, stored, and analyzed by friends and foes alike—no matter how unfairly—what is the hearing health care practitioner to do? Besides doing everything possible to safeguard your reputation and protect your bank account from identity thieves, here are two favorable outcomes that may be derived from Big Data and the Facebook Effect.

1. Better data-driven decisions. Practitioners can use the data collected from computerized office management systems to make better business decisions about their practice. For example, it is quite straightforward to construct a demand curve by taking a year or more of purchasing history in your practice, and then analyze the cost of goods sold and

the profit margins to better understand what devices and services need to be offered to more patients. From a clinical perspective these same office management systems could be used to evaluate possible correlations between outcomes and a wide range of procedures and best practices in the profession. Such an analysis could determine which procedures and practices are providing the biggest bang for the buck. Of course, this requires researchers to conduct (and the industry to fund) a lot more randomized clinical trials of hearing aids and their associated features and accessories.

2. Improve quality of care. Just as cameras and checklists in the operating room are reducing the rate of surgical complications, Big Data could do much the same for audiologists and hearing instrument dispensers. For example, relative benefit scores, results from satisfaction surveys, and return-for-credit rates for each clinic could be posted on websites of national organizations for everyone to see. Before a patient visits your clinic for a hearing evaluation, the person would already know how successful other patients have been. This would enable the consumer to make a truly informed choice based on quality of care and outcomes, rather than on marketing type and low price. AuDNet, a network of doctoral-level audiologists, has recently announced that it will provide better wholesale pricing to members who can demonstrate they use best practices and provide patients with the ability to rate their delivery of services. (AuDNet's Patient Care Excellence program checklist can be found in the Appendix.

@CONNECT

Atul Gawande

Atul Gawande, a leading proponent of health care reform, greater transparency, and quality initiatives, is a surgeon and author of several outstanding books, including *The Checklist Manifesto*. Visit his website at http://www.gawande.com for interesting articles and interviews.

In this age of patient-centered transparency, we can be hopeful that the cream will rise to the top and that the best clinicians will be generously rewarded for making data-driven decisions that drive both quality of care and profits. Are you ready for the change? Maybe this book will help.

Managing Change

Joseph Schumpeter (1883–1950), the Austrian-born economist, coined the term "creative destruction" to describe the method by which economic change occurred in a capitalist society. Schumpeter noted that the fundamental impulse that sets and keeps the capitalist engine in motion comes from new consumer goods, new methods of production, emerging markets, and new forms of industrial organization that entrepreneurs create. In Schumpeter's view of capitalism, entrepreneurs are the disruptive force that sustains economic progress.

Creative destruction and disruptive technology are all around us. If you were in the newspaper or recording industry 15 years ago, your profession has been thoroughly disrupted by the digital MP3 and tablet-computer goliaths. There is no reason to think that audiologists, hearing instrument specialists, physicians, and others involved in hearing care should be immune from the forces of creative destruction and disruptive innovation. The reality is that technology is getting so good and so cheap that many of the technical aspects of our job may soon be replaced by a machine. Just as the artisan weavers of the eighteenth century were replaced by the mechanical loom, audiologists may be replaced by computers that conduct accurate tests. A group called the Luddites fought the mechanization of textile production for decades, and lost. You have to wonder if it is worth fighting the disruptive forces in our profession.

The forces of creative destruction extend beyond disruptive technology per se. Other professions that once thought they were immune to the effects of outsourcing now find themselves marginalized by low-cost workers in Asia who speak good English and have advanced degrees in science and engineering. A physician in India can read x-rays and sonograms for a fraction of the cost of having them read by an American radiologist. The day may come when the troubleshooting and adjustment of hearing aids is done remotely from another country by professionals with advanced degrees.

Mass Customization

The previous two paragraphs illustrate a very narrow, technocentric view of the hearing care professions—one that some professionals do not agree with but that is widely held by many within the hearing care professions. While I commend the efforts of anyone willing to fight to maintain barriers to entry into our respective industry professions, I wonder if some of that energy could be better devoted to creatively engaging the marketplace in new and better ways of adding consumer value. Taking a page from Schumpeter, I propose that hearing care professionals of all stripes bring new services to market that cannot be replaced with technology or duplicated by lower cost outsourced labor. It is time to rally around the mass personalization of services.

There are three areas where the personalization of services by audiologists and hearing instrument specialists cannot be duplicated by machines or outsourced labor. All three of these personalized services require face-to-face interaction with a patient/customer:

1. Consultative selling: using evidence-based principles to identify a hearing loss and uncover an individualized solution. Once the patient's needs are identified, a solution is customized to their lifestyle and budget.
2. Personal adjustment counseling: working with a patient over a relatively extended period of time to unearth the emotional underpinnings of his or her hearing loss and helping the patient and family cope with it as they age. The foundation of personal adjustment counseling is motivational interviewing, which is covered in Chapter 3.
3. Individualized rehabilitation: working with patients to "retrain" their brain in the communication process and helping them become more proficient communicators.

When hearing care professionals are able to wrap a memorable and engaging experience around these three core competences, they will create value that cannot be duplicated by disruptive technology or outsourced labor. Capture the entrepreneurial experience and unleash the power of creative destruction in your practice.

@CONNECT

Joe Pine

One of the authors of the Experience Economy, Joe Pine is a leading authority on the concept of mass customization. Follow him on Twitter @joepine.

Value-Based Pricing Strategies

A chapter devoted to quality in the business suite would not be complete without a section on pricing and price strategy in a clinic. Let us examine the role of retail price in a practice and how it signals quality. Verbal communication, along with opposable thumbs, separates humans from the rest of the animal kingdom. When communication is compromised due to the loss of hearing, which is commonly associated with the aging process, individuals often seek the care and guidance of professionals. Audiologists and hearing-instrument specialists are uniquely equipped to help individuals suffering the effects of hearing impairment by offering customizable hearing aid fittings and expert support over a long period of time. These offerings, which usually comprise a labor-intensive process of tailoring a pair of devices to the impaired auditory system, plus patient counseling and guidance in the process of overcoming the effects of diminished communication as individuals age. Additionally, this comprehensive set of offerings has intrinsic value and its price is largely determined by market forces and next best alternatives, such as over-the-counter personal sound-amplification products, surgically implantable devices, or the patient's decision to do nothing. Let us examine *how* practitioners can unlock value in their offerings to these individuals suffering from the long-term effects of hearing loss using a value-based pricing strategy.

Confessions of an Over-Discounter

It is safe to say that audiologists do not learn too much in school about how to price their offerings. As a result, the profession suffers from a lack of autonomy, whereas patients, arguably, are restricted in their choices of service offerings. Before going any further, let me share my story as it relates to hearing aid pricing. There was a time early in my career when I thought lowering the price on the hearing aids I dispensed would lead to more sales. In order to gain agreement from patients, rather than defend the value of my recommendation, I found myself lowering the price on a specific technology tier or advising the patient to downgrade to a less expensive technology. As I have come to learn, hearing aids and their associated services exist in a largely inelastic market in which lowering the price does not translate into greater volumes of business. After reading further, I hope you do not repeat my mistakes.

My journey to better understanding how pricing and value effect the dispensing of hearing aids starts with some late-night television viewing. Like many others, I found myself temporarily mesmerized by the phenomenal deals on the Home Shopping Network. After all, who cannot use one of those gadgets that cooks your entire meal in 3 minutes! It might seem crass, but audiologists can learn a thing or two about how they price their products by watching infomercials. The legendary Ron Popeil of Ronco was the master of anchoring a high price point, demonstrating all of the cool features, reframing the product at a lower price to create a "wow" effect, and then restating an offer with value-added extras at a lower price. Even though audiology is a medically oriented profession, we oftentimes must have the resolve to ask people to pay large sums of money out-of-pocket for something they do not want. Ron Popeil offers insights on how to communicate price and value.

The purpose of this section is to discuss the importance of pricing strategy and the impact a carefully constructed pricing strategy has on both patient value and profitability of the business. Since hearing aid dispensing is a low-volume, high-margin business (since the market for hearing aids is quite small relative to other goods and services, it is considered a low-volume business that requires a significant amount of labor, and thus, relatively high margins are required to generate a profit), the prices we charge for these offerings take on greater importance relative to other businesses.

Let us continue our discussion of pricing strategy by asking ourselves a couple of critical questions. As you read this section, these questions should be on the top of your mind because the exact answer is highly dependent on your market, the competition, and how you differentiate your practice from competitors. Your thoughtful responses to these three overarching questions will help you formulate your "go-to-market" pricing strategy:

1. How do patients in your market benefit from your "product"? Product is in quotation marks because it represents both the devices and the service you deliver to ensure that the devices have been optimized to the patient's needs and expectations.
2. How is your "product" different than the competitor's next-best alternative on the market? For example, when it comes to hearing care services what other viable options are available to consumers in your marketplace? All of these options, from Internet distributors, a local ENT clinic—even doing nothing—are considered next best alternatives.
3. Does your clinic look and feel like a place where someone would willingly spend $10,000? This might seem like an inordinately high price, but that price tag will make sense toward the end of this section. As most of us have come to appreciate, the act of purchasing something has a strong emotional component and designing a practice that is emotionally appealing to the high end shopper has some inherent advantages.

Your responses to these questions require a deep dive into the values and mission of your practice. No two practices will answer them in the same way, and your answers will form the foundation for value-based pricing strategy in your clinic. Of course, you can expect the answers to the first two questions to be related to the devices you offer your patients, typically tiered along levels of technology varying by certain key features. In addition to the ubiquitous hearing aid device, there are several other attributes for which patients are willing to pay. These attributes include personalized service, prompt attention, expert guidance, peace of mind as a result of improved communication, ease of use, simplicity, and professional experience. Your task is to first construct a list of attributes that are unique to your practice relative to next best alternatives. Currently, most differentiation across practices and tiering of value is done almost exclusively with the device itself. Since the beginning of the digital-signal-processing era nearly 20 years ago, differentiation has been based on number of channels of wide dynamic range compression (WDRC). Not only is differentiation across technology based on channels lacking sufficient evidence (no more than 8 to 16 are needed to optimize audibility and sound quality), it ignores several other attributes that patients may value. Figure 5–5 contrasts two different pricing strategies. The pyramid on the left represents the traditional tiering of technology using channels of WDRC, whereas the pyramid on the right depicts a

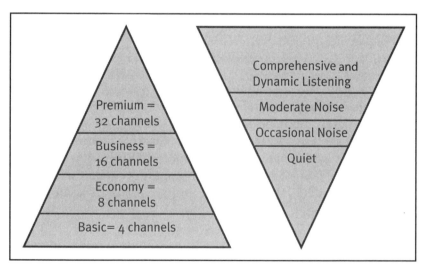

Figure 5–5. Traditional product tier based on number of channels of compression (*left*) versus tier driven by patient attributes.

more comprehensive method, incorporating other attributes that hearing-impaired customers and their families are more likely to value.

Let us examine some of the thinking behind the application of value-based pricing in a hearing aid dispensing practice. As previously mentioned, no one better exemplifies value-based price tactics than Ron Popeil of Ronco, which has put rotisserie ovens, pocket fisherman, and food dehydrators in millions of homes. What could clinicians possibly learn from Ronco? The answer is in how offerings are positioned to customers. There are three pricing tactics pioneered by Ron Popeil and mastered by infomercial producers for decades that can be readily applied to the pricing of hearing aids and their associated services:

1. Framing. The context in which a price is communicated to a customer effects how much the customer may be willing to pay. When a salesman such as Ron Popeil demonstrates a number of features, this is an example of framing. In the hearing aid market, audiologists could frame their offerings by demonstrating key features relative to alternatives that cost a lot more. For example, once the price and features of implantable hearing aids is shared with the patient, it helps frame a traditional pair of hearing aids at a lower price point.

   Another example of framing is the use of bundling (or unbundling) of your offerings. When many of the key technology and service features are itemized and a dollar value is assigned to each, it frames your offering much differently than if you were to simply list one price in a bundled format. Research has shown that unbundling results in many patients willing to pay more for the same offering (Amlani & Taylor, 2012). The concept of framing—the bundling and unbundling prices—is important to audiologists and receives more attention later.

2. Anchoring. Consumers have a pretty good idea of the value of products and services they purchase on a regular basis. For items you are used to buying (e.g., turkey on Thanksgiving, a new laptop computer, a gallon of milk, gasoline) you expect to pay a certain amount—these prices provide the anchors. If you see the offering listed for at a lower price, you may be more inclined to make a special trip to

the store to save some money. Anchoring is the reason why sales work so well. Based on their previous buying experience, customers know they are receiving a good deal when an especially low sale price is spotted in a newspaper ad or coupon. The problem associated with anchoring in the hearing aid market is that the average consumer is not too familiar with the time and expertise required to successfully fit the typical patient with hearing aids. When a dispensing practice runs advertising using low price points to drive traffic, an unintended consequence is anchoring that low price point in the mind of the prospective buyer. Once a price has been anchored, it is difficult to change the perception. That is why is it often very difficult to convince a "price shopper" that their long-term interests may be better served with a more sophisticated (and usually more expensive) offering.

3. Default bias. Consumers generally take a path of least resistance when making purchases. When an obstacle even as simple as checking a box to become eligible for a service or upgrade is placed in front of a customer, they oftentimes do not voluntarily opt for it. An example of the role default bias plays in markets is that of organ donations. In states that changed their organ-donation system from one that individuals had to opt into, to organ donation by checking a box during one's driver's license renewal, to a system in which individuals are automatically enrolled in the program unless they opted out by checking a box, the number of organ-donation volunteers more than doubled. Another good example of default bias at work comes from employer offered 401(k) retirement plans. When employees are automatically included in a 401(k) program, rather than having to voluntarily opt into the program, enrollment into the 401(k) program goes up dramatically. The lesson for audiologists with respect to default bias is that items that are necessary for the success of the patient need to be included in the price. These items may include a specific number of service visits over a finite period of time, extended warranties or even batteries. By allowing patients not to choose, they are more likely to get the services that are required to have long-term success with amplification.

FUNDAMENTALS OF SUPPLY AND DEMAND

Before getting into the details of value-based pricing strategy, let us continue our value-based pricing strategy journey by addressing some of the most fundamental concepts surrounding the buying and selling of common products. A good example of how changes in supply and demand change price can be found on a rainy day in New York City. Imagine you are attempting to walk from midtown Manhattan to Greenwich Village. As it begins to rain, you realize you do not have enough money for a taxi and you do not have time to navigate the gnarly subway system. Since your only choice is to walk without getting soaked, you spot the nearest street vendor with umbrellas for sale. As you approach his stand, you notice that he has raised the price of his umbrellas by $5. Since you do not want to get wet, his doubling of the umbrella price to $10 still seems like a pretty good deal.

To fully appreciate the laws of supply and demand and their relationship to price, let us examine this scenario two different ways. In the first scenario, let us say that the umbrella industry has lobbied the government to effectively restrict the number of licensed vendors who are able to sell umbrellas. The result of their lobbying efforts is that there are a limited number of vendors selling umbrellas (e.g., one vendor every 15 city blocks). This government action keeps the supply of umbrellas artificially low and, thus, the price relatively high. Restricting the number of vendors effectively keeps the competitors at bay, but it does not make all the rain-soaked customers very happy, as they either put up with paying the higher umbrella prices or seek alternatives, such as a newspaper to cover their head or a more expensive raincoat that is cumbersome to pack and use when rain starts to pour.

Now, let us look at umbrella usage in a free-market system where the high prices of umbrellas on a rainy day create incentives for entrepreneurs to enter the market and offer umbrellas at lower prices. In the free-market system, high prices are a signal to entrepreneurs that profits can be made by offering a next-best alternative at a lower price. Entrepreneurs who fail to compete with lower prices or a higher quality alternative priced higher are likely to be driven out of business. Of course, the customer ultimately wins in the free-market scenario because he has a range of choices as he walks through Manhattan on that rainy day. He can buy a really cheap umbrella that lasts for 1 day or one that is of much higher quality for more money that will last a lifetime, assuming he does not lose it. The free-market system represents greater choices for customers as well as increased opportunities for entrepreneurs to creatively address the needs of customers with unique product and service offerings. Value-based pricing strategies represent a method of unlocking these opportunities for both customers and entrepreneurs who serve the market.

Tyler Cowan and Alex Taborrek, economists at George Mason University, have coined the phrase "price is a signal wrapped in an incentive" to describe how pricing works in the real world. In the umbrella scenario price is a signal to customers and entrepreneurs alike. In a free-market system, it signals to entrepreneurs that profit opportunities exist, and for customers it signals that various choices of product are available at different price points. In addition to sending a signal, prices create incentives for customers to buy. As you will learn, value-based pricing strategy is predicated on your ability to recognize what various segments of your market value and find appealing about your offering, and creating incentives for those customers to purchase from you.

Traditionally, most practices use either a simple markup or a margin-based pricing strategy. The simplest of the two is a mark-up strategy. With a simple markup strategy, the manager applies a multiplier to the wholesale cost to obtain the retail cost. For example, if your markup is 100%, the wholesale cost is multiplied by two to get the retail price. A margin-based pricing is slightly more sophisticated, however, as more attention is paid to keeping the whole cost of goods of all products in alignment with the cost of running the business. For example, in a purely margin-based strategy, the manager determines the cost of goods required to maintain a specific gross profit that is needed to maintain a sustainable business. Both strategies are dependent on the practice manager doing some breakeven cost evaluations to ensure that they are charging enough to cover costs and make a marginal profit, so they can stay in business. The one thing lacking in both the margin-based and simple markup strategy is a detailed analysis on what attributes are desired by different segments of the market, and how prices can be presented to unlock that value across various customer segments. The three types of pricing strategy are summarized in Table 5–4.

Value-Based Pricing Strategy

Margin-based and simple mark-up pricing strategies require you to think like an accountant. On the other hand, the key to understanding value-based pricing is thinking like a customer. Since all of us buy things just about every day, it should not be too difficult to think like one. The attributes of the products and services we buy determine its value. This forms the basis for value-based pricing. Characteristics such as price, convenience, performance, and simplicity determine how much customers are willing to pay for something. The more we value a certain attribute, the more we are willing to pay for it. Value-based pricing is used to sell multiple offerings at multiple prices by identifying the key attributes for which customers are willing to pay more or less. According to Mohammed (2010) value-based pricing is a five-step process involving:

1. Identifying target customers
2. Identifying their next best alternatives
3. Determining your offering's differences
4. Calculating your offering's value based on its differentiation
5. Making sure your pricing is competitive and reality based.

Table 5–4. The Three Types of Pricing Strategy

Simple markup
Margin based
Value based

A quick example might help to better understand value-based pricing strategy using this five-step process. Let us say that you have a 1973 Porsche convertible. It is a relatively rare car in mint condition. Mohammed's five steps can be used to determine your asking price. First, you might spend some time carefully identifying your target market and you might make the decision to advertise on websites that cater to men over the age of 50 years, because you believe that this segment of the population finds such vintage cars most appealing and would have the discretionary income to buy one. Second, you would evaluate the next-best alternatives on the market. In this example, next-best alternatives might include new sports cars and other similar vintage sports coupes listed on Craig's List. Third, you would determine the attributes of the car that are unusual, rare, or highly valued by certain segments of your market. In the case of the Porsche, this would be that it is a convertible and that it a hard to find red color. Because these attributes are rare, you will be able to charge more for them. Fourth, you would calculate the asking price based on these differences relative to the results of steps two and three. Maybe you have found that people are willing to pay an extra 25% for vintage convertible roadsters. This allows you to price the car at a higher price with the confidence that there are a pool of interested buyers ready to hand you a certified bank check for it. Finally, after you have established a price for the car, you do some double-checking to make sure your price is consistent with comparable cars that are on the market. For example, if your preliminary price is several hundred dollars higher than the next highest price, you may consider dropping your asking price slightly.

Notice that a true value-based pricing strategy, like the example above, is not a simple markup of the wholesale price or based on a margin percent. Rather, a value-based strategy, in its purest form, relies on the seller to carefully calibrate the needs of the market and the attributes of the product to determine the asking price. The five-step value-based pricing strategy above works well for selling one product in relatively high demand, but can the strategy be effectively employed with hearing aids? Following some reality-based guidelines with a few modifications, value-based pricing can be used to establish retail prices in your clinic.

Before we tackle a value-based pricing strategy, however, let us spend some time reviewing some of the nuances of the hearing aid dispensing business that make it different from selling a cherry red vintage Porsche. The hearing aid dispensing market is unique for a number of reasons cited previously:

1. Because there are a relatively small number of buyers for hearing aid services compared with other products, practitioners must maintain relatively high margins in order to make a profit and stay in business. Brady (2010) uses a concept called the "Rule of Thirds" to calculate the cost of goods and gross profit needed to cover expenses and make a pretax profit. Using Brady's rule, the cost of goods needs to be around 30 to 35% of the retail cost of the offering to each patient. Maintaining this cost-of-goods range requires practitioners to be strong negotiators with their vendor partners and to thoroughly evaluate the price charged to patients.

2. Lowering the prices you charge does not increase total volume. Amlani (2009) showed that lowering the retail price does not have an appreciable effect on demand. This indicates that the hearing aid market is relatively inelastic, as his work suggests that demand does not change for prices between $500 and $3,000 per unit. As the provocative title of Amlani's 2009 article suggests, practitioners are not immoral when they raise their prices; thus, they must look for ways to build value into their offerings without lowering retail prices.

3. Recent MarkeTrak survey data indicate that approximately one third of hearing aid purchases are reimbursed or covered by third-party payers, such as health insurance companies. Depending on the patient's specific medical plan, the costs are covered either completely or partially. Partial coverage of hearing aids represents a partial incentive, as the patient is required to pay the difference out-of-pocket if he or she wants to upgrade. The work of Ramachandran, Stach, and Becker (2011) suggests that these partial incentives do not work. In their study they evaluated the product level, age of acquisition, and degree of hearing loss of three groups: full coverage of hearing aids, partial coverage of hearing aids, and out-of-pocket private pay. Their findings showed that full coverage lowered the age of acquisition and attracted

patients with milder hearing loss, whereas partial coverage does not. Moreover, their findings indicated that patients with partial coverage were less likely to upgrade to higher levels of technology or wear a bilateral hearing aid arrangement relative to both the full-coverage and private-pay cohorts. This study indicates to practitioners that (1) partial coverage does not incentivize a patient to upgrade very often by paying the out-of-pocket difference, and (2) there is a relatively strong private-pay market for midlevel and premium offerings—even in the presence of full- and partial-coverage insurance offerings.

4. As previously mentioned, how you talk price determines a customer's willingness to pay. This concept is known as framing. When features are unbundled and assigned a dollar value, customers are willing to pay more than when the offering components are bundled together and sold at one flat price. Amlani, Taylor, and Weinberg (2011) showed three groups of retired adults three hearing aid advertisements. All groups were shown the same hearing aid, but each of the three ads had a different written message accompanying it. Group 1 was shown the ad with very little information pertaining to features, group 2 was shown a feature-laden ad, and group 3 was shown an ad that was benefit driven. The ads shown to groups 2 and 3 were considered unbundled, as key features and benefits were listed as individual bullet points. Results indicated that patients who were shown the unbundled messages were willing to pay slightly more for the same device. Furthermore, Amlani et al. (2011) indicated that experienced hearing aid users were willing to pay more when technical benefits were unbundled, while inexperienced hearing aid users were willing to pay more when nontechnical service-oriented features were unbundled and assigned an individual dollar value. Taken as a whole, the work of Amlani et al. (2011) suggest that unbundling product and service benefits tend to increase patients' willingness-to-pay. Unbundling service and product attributes may enhance perceived value over a completely bundled approach. The challenge for practitioners is knowing what product and service benefits to unbundle. This is addressed later in this chapter.

What Attributes Do Customers Value Most?

This section provides practitioners with a template for implementing a customized version of a value-based pricing strategy for their own clinic. Before delving into those details, let us briefly examine a topic of relatively recent interest, which is the unbundling of prices. As a general rule, practitioners in the hearing aid industry have traditionally bundled their offerings to consumers. This means that several features and services are combined (or bundled) and offered to patients at a single price point. For example, the practitioner might bundle the hearing evaluation, hearing aid fitting fee, hearing aid, and warranty into a single unit price. The chief advantage of bundling is simplicity. Because patients are given a single price with several benefits wrapped into one flat fee, it is believed that customers are more apt to make a purchasing decision (Tjan, 2010).

Over the past few years, unbundling has gained popularity among practitioners, especially those in private practice. In an unbundling format many of the key attributes of the offering are itemized and a dollar value is assigned for each of them. For the consumer, unbundling offers them an "a la carte" selection of product and service offerings. For the practitioner, unbundling has the potential to increase revenue for various clinical procedures that otherwise might have been bundled into the price of the hearing aid itself. Unbundling likely has become a more popular strategy by practitioners because more third-party insurers are able to reimburse for various procedures that are completed during the hearing aid selection and fitting process. Additionally, Sjoblad and Warren (2001) have suggested that unbundling allows practices an opportunity to show the value of various clinical procedures by assigning a dollar value to them that is separate from the price of the device itself. Although unbundling represents greater potential revenue opportunities for practice owners, experts suggest that it allows customers an opportunity to negotiate for services that are a necessary component of their comprehensive care (Tjan, 2010). Although there are no studies that have directly compared the revenue generated using an unbundled versus a bundled pricing model, anecdotal evidence suggests that a purely unbundled pricing model leads to greater generation of revenue from testing, but also leads to more haggling over some of the necessary components of long-term patient care. Perhaps balance is needed between the benefits of unbundling and bundling of offerings that benefits the long-term care needs of the patient along with the revenue needs of the practice.

In order to balance the needs of patients to receive a high-quality service experience with those of the practice to optimize revenues that keep the business sustainable, a hybrid approach to pricing strategy that takes the best elements of both the unbundled and bundled models is needed. For practices looking to optimize revenue while maintaining high standards of comprehensive patient care, the following four-step value-based pricing strategy is proposed.

1. Cost and margin analysis. Using the principles put forth by Coverstone (2012), Brady (2010), and Sjoblad and Warren (2011), practices must carefully evaluate the current cost of goods, fixed and variable costs, as well as break-even points. This requires a detailed analysis of current cost of goods and gross profit for each hearing aid dispensed over the past year. Once current costs and margins are understood, the practice must work to bring the cost of goods to between 30% and 35% across all technology tiers. Figure 5–6 is an example of how the cost of goods and gross profit looks under such a tiered system. Note there are four price points in this simplified tiered approach and the gross profit margin (retail price minus cost of goods) is known for each tier.

2. Obtain customer feedback. The second step requires that practices use the best available data to construct a simple demand curve. In larger corporations a demand curve is constructed using sophisticated market-research analysis in order to evaluate the demand for particular products and features at various price points. Ulwick (2005) charted various products on a four-quadrant matrix based on emotional and functional complexity. Figure 5–7 shows that medical devices are rated solidly in the functional complexity category. Ulwick's work implies that the tiering of hearing aid technology should be based on functional complexity. In other words, as the functionality becomes more sophisticated, the price increases. Clearly, the common practice of

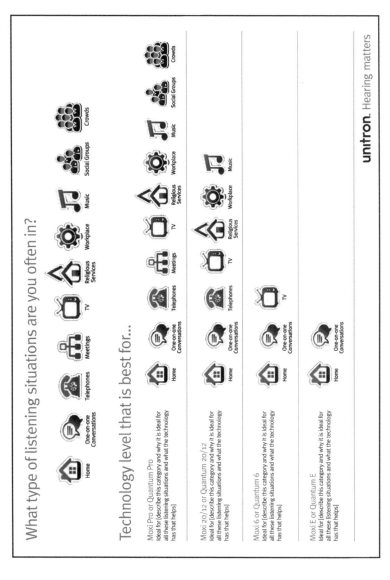

Figure 5–6. An example of COGs and gross profit using a tiered approach to price strategy for a hypothetical practice.

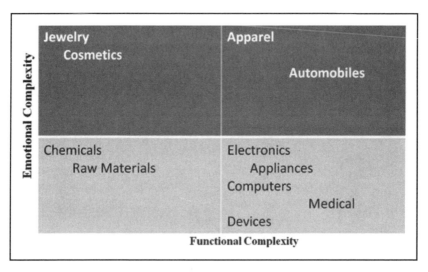

Figure 5–7. Four-quadrant matrix based on emotional and functional complexity. (From Ulwick, 2005)

tiering hearing aid technology based purely on number of channels does not fully leverage Ulwick's model.

For the private practice this type of market analysis is not readily available. The good news, however, is that practices can rely on simpler methods to help establish value-based price points. A combination of past buying history in their own practice and published research from the hearing aid industry can be used to establish the attributes of your offerings across various price points. Both MarkeTrak VI, and Bridges, Lataille, Buttorff, White, and Niparko (2012), indicated that performance in background is the primary attribute sought by hearing aid users. This was followed by improved sound quality, feedback reduction, and comfort. Knowledge of the chief attributes sought by hearing aid users can be used in creating your value-based pricing system. As Figure 5–6 suggests, as you move up the tiers, the attributes that are most important for the buyer increase in technological sophistication as well as price. The tiering of hearing aid prices based on technical attributes is geared mainly toward experienced users of amplification. As Amlani et al. (2011) suggest, inexperienced hearing aid users are likely to value many of the nontechnical attributes, such as service and warranty. This represents an opportunity to tier service attributes as well. Performance in background noise, automatic and wireless features, and various levels of warranty and service represent some of the opportunities to tier value at three to four distinct price points.

3. Tier attributes at specific price points. Once you have done the preliminary work of evaluating margins and costs, and you have obtained some voice-of-customer information about attributes that are most valued, it is time to formalize your go-to-market offerings at three of four tiered prices. For instructional purposes, let us say our hypothetical practice has decided to create three distinct offerings at three price points: $2,000, $3,500, and $5,000. The first step is to establish your baseline or entry-level offering by asking yourself what the minimum technology and service offerings are that you are willing to provide for all of your patients. For example, your margin-and-cost analysis indicates that you can profitably provide to the market a $2,000 entry-level offer. What features and services do you provide at this price point? Table 5–5 shows an example of features and benefits that can be offered at an entry-level price of $2,000. Readers should note that the tiers presented in this chapter are examples and individual versions of itemized bundles will vary depending on market forces and other variables.

Table 5–5. Example of Tiered Pricing Strategy Following Analysis of Cost of Goods

Patient Price/Unit	Wholesale Price/Unit[a]	Cost of Goods (%)	Margin/Gross Profit per Device[b]
$2,800	$924	33	$1,874
$2,345	$750	32	$1,595
$1,485	$475	32	$1,010
$995	$328	33	$667

[a]Price includes 2-year warranty.
[b]List prices do not include hearing evaluation or fitting fee.

Once you have establish your baseline tier or package (Table 5–6), the next step is to devise one or two additional tiers that will comprise your midlevel offering. In the midlevel tiers the attributes that are typically valued the most by customers, such as more sophisticated technology for hearing in background noise, automatic features, and more comprehensive or longer service packages, are built into the midlevel offering. Table 5–7 represents an example of a midlevel offering. The critical question would be, is this offering worth an additional $1,500 to the patient?

The final step is to create a premium offering at the highest price point. This can be done by adding to the attributes valued the most by customers. Table 5–8 is an example of value-added attributes at the premium level. As you create the premium package, the critical issue is insuring that it has a perceived value to the patient of an additional $1,500 relative to the midlevel offering.

Table 5–6. Baseline Package

Two devices designed for listening mainly in quiet environments (no automatic features or wireless accessories)
One-year service package (unlimited office visits)
One-year warranty
Availability of aural rehabilitation classes or auditory training

Table 5–7. Midlevel Package

Two devices designed for listening in moderate amounts of background noise with a limited number of automatic processing features
One wireless accessory
Two-year service package (unlimited office visits)
Two-year warranty
Availability of aural rehabilitation classes or auditory training

Table 5–8. Premium Package

Two devices designed for listening in complex listening environments with a significant amount of automatic processing (e.g., beam-forming directional microphones)

Two wireless accessories

Two-year service package (unlimited office visits)

Two-year warranty

Availability of aural rehabilitation classes or auditory training

The goal of creating tiers or packages at three or four specific price points is to strike a balance between a relatively limited amount of choices to customers and offering a number of attributes valued the most by customers. Moreover, as you will recall from the summary of default bias earlier in this chapter, practitioners can build features into each tier or package that will lead to more favorable outcomes. For example, making a year of office visits part of the bundle is likely to incentivize patients to come in for office visits when there is a problem or question. This value-based approach is a hybrid that takes the advantages of both a bundled and unbundled strategy. This approach is known as versioning (Mohammed, 2010) because it combines several attributes into three or four packages from which customers can choose.

4. Signal to the market with itemized bundles. The compromise between purely unbundled and bundled offerings is best explained as an itemized bundle approach. In an itemized bundle approach, practitioners are able to unbundle the necessary testing procedures that need to be completed on each patient prior to purchasing hearing aids. Procedures that may in fact be reimbursable by third-party payers. Unbundling these required procedures shows the value of these essential diagnostic procedures, whereas bundling all other components of offerings across three or four tiers gives the patient some simple choices (versions) from which to choose. Using itemized bundles makes it unlikely that

they will haggle over necessary components of the offering because they have been bundled into the price (Tjan, 2010). An example of an itemized bundle is shown in Table 5–9 for a midlevel offering. Note that the patient is responsible for paying the dispensing and evaluation fee, but the rest of the offering is bundled together. The $100 hearing evaluation fee and the $200 consultation fee could be submitted to a third-party payer for reimbursement or the patient could pay out-of-pocket. The total cost for the itemized bundle shown in Table 5–9 is $3,800.

Using itemized bundles, such as the example shown in Table 5–9, enables practices to strike a balance between value and simplicity. By unbundling the prefitting procedures, practices are able to demarcate their value for specific test procedures needed to identify type and degree of hearing loss while also obtaining reimbursement from third-party payers when possible. At the same time, bundling many of the features required for a successful fitting keeps the number of patient choices at a manageable level.

In addition to the itemized-bundle "versioning" strategy, there are two other value-based pricing strategy tactics outlined

Table 5–9. Example of an Itemized Bundle with Three Separate Fees

Hearing evaluation: $100
Dispensing/consultation fee: $200
Two devices designed for listening in moderate amounts of background noise with a modest amount of automatic processing
One wireless accessory
Two-year service package (unlimited office visits)
Two-year warranty
Availability of aural rehabilitation classes or auditory training
Midlevel package: $3,500

by Mohammed (2010) that may have utility in a hearing aid dispensing practice:

- Pick-a-plan. Internet distributors and third-party payers oftentimes enable practitioners to collect a professional fitting fee for their service time. From a value-based price strategy perspective, this represents a pick-a-plan tactic. Although perhaps not as profitable to the business, using a pick-a-plan tactic can attract a different segment of the hearing aid market to your practice that you ordinarily would not see in a personalized service business: the price-conscious shopper.
- Differential pricing. The use of coupons, club memberships, and subscriptions are examples of differential pricing tactics (Mohammed, 2010). Differential pricing can be used to bridge the gaps between the itemized bundles discussed previously. For example, a practice could create an "a la carte" menu of items such as assistive devices, wireless accessories, and sundry items that are offered to patients. If an individual decided to purchase the "Advanced Bundle" but really needed an assistive device for television viewing, they could be guided to purchase something from the "a la carte" menu. Differential pricing tactics can also be employed for capturing business from the public-assistance market. Depending on the funding source, practices can use differential pricing tactics to create incentives by offering basic digital technology at a low price point.

HIGH PRICE SIGNALS HIGH QUALITY

If price is a signal your practice sends to the market, then given the high price points paid out-of-pocket relative to other offerings in the health care arena, audiologists are definitely sending a signal of high quality. The essential question is, does your practice exude high quality and look like a place where people would be willing to spend upward of $10,000? It is only through the foundation of a culture devoted to continuous improvement, judicious use of best practices, and dedication to creating a remarkable patient experience that this will occur. Using a value-based pricing strategy is simply your signal to the market that your practice represents these characteristics. By offering itemized bundles across three to four price points that list comprehensive services and technology tiered to the most attributes customers value the most (primarily performance in background noise and personalized service), practices can signal to a wide segment of the market using itemized bundles. This approach represents the next-best alternative to a slew of direct-to-consumer and run-of-the-mill, mediocre service providers. As Ron Popeil says, "Now, wait, there's more." For audiologists his quote signals an opportunity to differentiate their offerings from numerous low-end competitors.

GETTING THE RIGHT STUFF DONE

Quality in the business suite requires managers, owners, and clinicians to juggle many items simultaneously. In reality, this boils down to establishing clear priorities and devising actionable strategies devoted to continuous improvement. With continuous improvement being one of the cornerstones of quality, let us review a process that allows all the stakeholders in a practice to thrive. Anyone who has been in a busy clinic or practice knows that there is a lot of bustle associated with the demands of seeing patients. It is sometimes nearly impossible to step away from this storm of daily activity to make improvements in your practice; however, a culture devoted to quality demands that we do something every day to try and improve gaps associated with patient care and business management. Here is a four-step process that can be adapted by practitioners in order to get your strategic priorities off the ground:

- ■ Step 1: Set one big goal. Identify one activity that results in optimizing patient care or increasing practice revenue. Only one at a time! An example might be to improve the quality of hearing aid evaluation appointments.

- Step 2: Implement standards using lead measures as your gauge. Using best practice guidelines, educate your staff on all the essential behaviors that must be engaged with the patient. Use one lead measure to monitor progress. For the reasons cited previously, it is necessary for this to be a *lead* measure, since lead measures give insight into future results and can be acted upon quickly. For the example in step 1, a lead measure might be the number of patients agreeing to purchase hearing aids who are true candidates for them. Along with your lead measure, make sure you have a benchmark or goal that you are trying to achieve, and a time line for when you expect to reach this benchmark or goal.
- Step 3: Monitor lead measures. Each week or month look at the KPIs report of the lead measure you have created. Review it with staff and decide what actions, if any, need to be completed.
- Step 4: Create a rhythm surrounding ongoing activity. Work with your staff to identify a time when the entire team can meet to review KPIs reports and lead measures. Work together to establish changes in workflow or standards that are required to better meet your one goal. Allow staff to try new things and report on how it went with respect to the goal. Once the gap has been sufficiently closed on one goal, create another goal.

WHAT QUALITY LOOKS LIKE

Next to a car, hearing aids are the most expensive item many people over the age of 70 years will purchase. For this reason alone we owe it to our patients to infuse our practices with quality. Applying the principles outlined in this text, practitioners can reap the rewards of quality and excellence as competitive advantages. Among these advantages are more word-of-mouth referrals and maintaining a higher than average selling price for your offerings.

At the heart of quality are several core principles that must be embraced by all staff members. The best restaurants, sports teams, and health care facilities all do the following:

- Create a culture committed to excellence and incremental self-improvement
- Orchestrate staff to play specific roles within the business
- Follow best practice standards that create consistently strong habits
- Inspect standards so that the entire staff is accountable for outcomes
- Listen to feedback from customers in order to make data-driven decisions
- Act on feedback in a prioritized and deliberate manner in order to incrementally improve outcomes.

In a hearing aid dispensing or audiology practice the delivery mechanism for providing this service is the six-step patient experience model. By centering the delivery of services around a memorable theme using memorabilia when appropriate, practitioners are able to clearly differentiate their offerings. By integrating the quality principles in this book, you can use the following template to stage the six essential "touch points" of the patient experience in your practice:

1. Promotion/Awareness

   A. Key behaviors/best practices required to deliver:

   B. Memorabilia and signature moments that tie to your theme:

2. Phone Scheduling

   A. Key behaviors/best practices required to deliver:

   B. Memorabilia and signature moments that tie to your theme:

3. Greeting and Waiting Room Experience

   A. Key behaviors/best practices required to deliver:

   B. Memorabilia and signature moments that tie to your theme:

4. Testing and Recommendation

   A. Key behaviors/best practices required to deliver:

   B. Memorabilia and signature moments that tie to your theme:

5. Fitting and Purchase

   A. Key behaviors/best practices required to deliver:

   B. Memorabilia and signature moments that tie to your theme:

6. Follow-Up

   A. Key behaviors/best practices required to deliver:

   B. Memorabilia and signature moments that tie to your theme:

REFERENCES

Amlani, A. (2009) It's not immoral to increase hearing aid prices in an inelastic market. *Hearing Review*, *18*(13), 10–17.

Amlani, A., & Taylor, B. (2012). Three known factors that impede hearing aid adoption rates. *Hearing Review*, *19*(5), 28–37.

Brady, G. (2010). Pricing for profit: How to set realistic profit margins. *Audiology Online*. Retrieved February 25, 2013.

Bridges, J., Lataille, A. T., Buttorff, C., White, S., & Niparko, J. K. (2012). Consumer preferences for hearing aid attributes: A comparison of rating and conjoint analysis methods. *Trends in Amplification, 16*(1), 40–48.

Carter, S. L. (1997). *Integrity.* New York, NY: Basic Books.

Coverstone, J. (2012). 20Q: Fee for service in an audiology practice. *Audiology Online.* Retrieved February 25, 2012

Crabtree, G. (2011). *Simple numbers, straight talk, big profits.* Austin, TX: Greenleaf Press.

Mahdavi, S. (2010). Seven rules for thinking about hearing aid pricing. *Hearing Review, 17*(9), 26–38.

Mohammed, R. (2010). *The 1% windfall: How successful companies use price to profit and grow.* New York, NY: Harper Business.

Ramachandran, V., Stach, B., & Becker, E. (2011). Reducing hearing aid cost does not influence device acquisition for milder hearing loss, but eliminating it does. *Hearing Journal, 64*(5), 10–18.

Sjoblad, S., & Warren, B. W. (2011). Can you unbundle and stay in business? *Audiology Today, 25*(5), 36–45.

Tjan, T. (2010). *The pros and cons of bundled pricing.* HBR blog. Retrieved February 26, 2010.

Ulwick, A. (2005). *What customers want: Using outcome-driven innovation to create breakthrough products and services.* New York, NY: McGraw-Hill.

APPENDIX

One of the cornerstones of quality is an ability to take decisive action once you have gathered some data and brainstormed possible causes to a gap in performance or outcomes. With that in mind, you may find from time to time that the worksheets, surveys, and other assorted items in this Appendix are helpful tools. Feel free to use them in your pursuit of quality in your clinic or office.

For each of the six interaction stations or segments of the patient journey listed below, use the worksheet to devise a plan for implementing them in your practice around a unifying theme. Work with your staff to complete the worksheet for each of the six interaction stations. This worksheet will help you get from A to almost Z.

1. Promotion/Awareness
2. Initial Phone Interaction
3. In-Office Greeting/Waiting Room
4. Testing/Recommendation
5. Fitting/Purchase
6. Follow-Up

QUALITY PATIENT EXPERIENCE WORKSHEET

1. Promotion/Awareness

    A. What is the sequence of behaviors needed to perform this with excellence (list below)?

    B. What tools (memorabilia, equipment, etc.) are needed to tie this interaction station with the overall theme or impression I am trying to make with each patient?

    C. What key performance indicators will measure the successful execution of these behaviors?

    D. How often will the staff review key performance indicators and quality process?

2. Initial Phone Interaction

    A. What is the sequence of behaviors needed to perform this with excellence (list below)?

B. What tools (memorabilia, equipment, etc.) are needed to tie this interaction station with the overall theme or impression I am trying to make with each patient?

C. What key performance indicators will measure the successful execution of these behaviors?

D. How often will the staff review key performance indicators and quality process?

3. In-office Greeting/Waiting Room

A. What is the sequence of behaviors needed to perform this with excellence (list below)?

B. What tools (memorabilia, equipment, etc.) are needed to tie this interaction station with the overall theme or impression I am trying to make with each patient?

C. What key performance indicators will measure the successful execution of these behaviors?

D. How often will the staff review key performance indicators and quality process?

4. Testing/Recommendation

A. What is the sequence of behaviors needed to perform this with excellence (list below)?

B. What tools (memorabilia, equipment, etc.) are needed to tie this interaction station with the overall theme or impression I am trying to make with each patient?

C. What key performance indicators will measure the successful execution of these behaviors?

D. How often will the staff review key performance indicators and quality process?

5. Fitting/Purchase

    A. What is the sequence of behaviors needed to perform this with excellence (list below)?

    B. What tools (memorabilia, equipment, etc.) are needed to tie this interaction station with the overall theme or impression I am trying to make with each patient?

    C. What key performance indicators will measure the successful execution of these behaviors?

    D. How often will the staff review key performance indicators and quality process?

6. Follow-Up

    A. What is the sequence of behaviors needed to perform this with excellence (list below)

B. What tools (memorabilia, equipment, etc.) are needed to tie this interaction station with the overall theme or impression I am trying to make with each patient?

C. What key performance indicators will measure the successful execution of these behaviors?

D. How often will the staff review key performance indicators and quality process?

EARTRAK SURVEY

EarTrak, an Australian company, offers a good example of a patient questionnaire that measures satisfaction with product and service quality. They have generously allowed us to reprint the entire questionnaire here. To learn more about EarTrak's questionnaire and report system you can contact Susan Clutterbuck at the following address:

Susan Clutterbuck
EARtrak pty ltd
ABN 70 112 449 555
PO Box 595
Traralgon VIC 3844
Australia
Phone: +61 3 5174 0699
Fax: +61 3 5174 8267
E-mail: outcomes@eartrak.com

Practice #	Client #

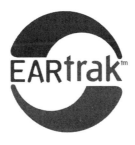

Survey of client opinion

Thank you for taking a few minutes to answer these questions which will help to improve hearing services. There is also room for you to record any comments you may wish to make. (Mark your answers with an "X")

Please rate your degree of difficulty when you are <u>not</u> wearing a hearing aid.

none	mild	moderate	moderate to severe	severe
☐	☐	☐	☐	☐

1. Over the last 2 weeks, how many **hours** on average did you use your hearing aid(s)?

none	less than 1 hour a day	1 to 4 hours a day	4 to 8 hours a day	more than 8 hours a day
☐	☐	☐	☐	☐

2. Think about the situations where you most wanted to hear better, before you got your present hearing aid(s).
Over the past two weeks, how much has the hearing aid **helped** in that situation?

helped not at all	helped slightly	helped moderately	helped quite a lot	helped very much
☐	☐	☐	☐	☐

3. Think again about the situation where you most wanted to hear better. When you use your present hearing aid(s), how much difficulty do you **STILL have** in that situation?

very much difficulty	quite a lot of difficulty	moderate difficulty	slight difficulty	no difficulty
☐	☐	☐	☐	☐

4. Considering everything, do you think your present hearing aid(s) **worth the trouble?**

not at all worth it	slightly worth it	moderately worth it	quite a lot worth it	very much worth it
☐	☐	☐	☐	☐

5. Over the past two weeks, with your present hearing aid(s), how much have your hearing difficulties affected **the things you do?**

affected very much	affected quite a lot	affected moderately	affected slightly	affected not at all
☐	☐	☐	☐	☐

6. Over the past two weeks, with your present hearing aid(s), how much do you think **other people** were bothered by your hearing difficulties?

bothered very much	bothered quite a lot	bothered moderately	bothered slightly	bothered not at all
☐	☐	☐	☐	☐

7. Considering everything, how much has your present hearing aid(s) changed your **enjoyment of life?**

worse	no change	slightly better	quite a lot better	very much better
☐	☐	☐	☐	☐

Please turn the page

8. Overall, **how satisfied** are you with your hearing aid(s)?

very dissatisfied	dissatisfied	neutral	satisfied	very satisfied
☐	☐	☐	☐	☐

9. Would you **recommend hearing aids** to a friend or family member with a hearing problem?

no	not sure	yes
☐	☐	☐

10. Would you **recommend your hearing service provider** to a friend or relative with a hearing problem?

no	not sure	yes
☐	☐	☐

11. How did you learn about your hearing service provider?

Doctor	Friend/ relative	Yellow pages	TV/ radio	News-paper	Work-place	Government Agency	Internet
☐	☐	☐	☐	☐	☐	☐	☐

Other -
Please specify

12. Listed below are some **listening situations**. Please mark **how satisfied** you are with your current hearing aid(s) for each situation. (Mark your answers with an "X" on each line). The term 'neutral' means neither satisfied nor dissatisfied.

Listening situation	not relevant	very dissatisfied	dissatisfied	neutral	satisfied	very satisfied
conversation with one person	☐	☐	☐	☐	☐	☐
in small groups	☐	☐	☐	☐	☐	☐
in large groups	☐	☐	☐	☐	☐	☐
outdoors	☐	☐	☐	☐	☐	☐
concert/movie	☐	☐	☐	☐	☐	☐
place of worship/lectures	☐	☐	☐	☐	☐	☐
watching TV	☐	☐	☐	☐	☐	☐
in a car	☐	☐	☐	☐	☐	☐
workplace	☐	☐	☐	☐	☐	☐
telephone	☐	☐	☐	☐	☐	☐
restaurant	☐	☐	☐	☐	☐	☐

If you would like to make any comments about **listening with your hearing aid(s)**, please write them here.

_____
_____
_____
_____
_____

Please turn the page

13. Listed below are some **hearing aid features**. Please mark **how satisfied** you are with each feature. (Mark your answers with an "X" on each line) The term 'neutral' means neither satisfied nor dissatisfied.

Hearing Aid Feature	not relevant	very dissatisfied	dissatisfied	neutral	satisfied	very satisfied
overall fit/ comfort	☐	☐	☐	☐	☐	☐
ease of adjusting volume	☐	☐	☐	☐	☐	☐
visibility of hearing aid	☐	☐	☐	☐	☐	☐
frequency of cleaning required	☐	☐	☐	☐	☐	☐
ongoing expense (eg. batteries, maintenance)	☐	☐	☐	☐	☐	☐
battery life	☐	☐	☐	☐	☐	☐
reliability	☐	☐	☐	☐	☐	☐
clarity of tone and sound	☐	☐	☐	☐	☐	☐
sound of own voice	☐	☐	☐	☐	☐	☐
ability to tell location of sounds	☐	☐	☐	☐	☐	☐
comfort with loud sounds	☐	☐	☐	☐	☐	☐
whistling/ feedback/buzzing	☐	☐	☐	☐	☐	☐

If you have **any comments about your hearing aid(s)**, please write them here. (Include an extra sheet if you want to write more than this space allows. We are interested in *all* of your comments.)

_____

_____

14. Listed below are some **features of your hearing service provider**. Please mark **how satisfied** you are with each aspect of the service. (Mark your answers with an "X" on each line). The term 'neutral' means neither satisfied nor dissatisfied.

Service Feature	very dissatisfied	dissatisfied	neutral	satisfied	very satisfied
Professionalism of clinician	☐	☐	☐	☐	☐
Friendliness of staff	☐	☐	☐	☐	☐
Patience of clinician	☐	☐	☐	☐	☐
Explanations given to you	☐	☐	☐	☐	☐
Amount of time spent with you	☐	☐	☐	☐	☐
Cleanliness and appearance of the office	☐	☐	☐	☐	☐
Quality of service after purchase	☐	☐	☐	☐	☐
Clinician understood my needs	☐	☐	☐	☐	☐

If you have **any comments about the service you've experienced,** please write them here. (Include an extra sheet if you want to write more than this space allows. We are interested in *all* of your comments.)

_____
_____
_____
_____
_____
_____
_____
_____
_____
_____
_____

Please turn the page

Your comments are important to your service provider.
Do you want us to send your comments to your service provider?

☐ Yes

☐ No

Do you want to be contacted by your service provider?

☐ Yes, I'd like to be contacted soon to review my fitting

☐ Yes, but only for routine rechecks

☐ No, I'll contact the provider if necessary

THANK YOU!

Please return your survey in the enclosed envelope.

Ref: 012

AUDNET PATIENT EXCELLENCE GUIDELINES

The group AudNet (http://www.aud-net.com) launched a patient excellence program that allows AuDNet members to receive an additional 2% discount if they follow best practice standards and agree to have their patients' satisfaction levels routinely surveyed and reported to the industry. Dave Smriga, President of AuDNet, has allowed us to reprint their patient excellence guidelines. It is a fantastic example of creating incentives around best practices and transparency, which are both pillars of quality.

Patient Care Excellence Discount Program Details

Program Components: Drafted from American Academy of Audiology. (2006). Audiologic Management of Adult Hearing Impairment—Summary Guidelines." *Audiology Today*, *18*(5), 33–36.

Initial "Patient Care Excellence" Disclosure Contract

Individual AuDNet member practices (or practices who are considering becoming members of AuDNet) will read and sign a contract indicating:

1. The patient care procedures they are agreeing to provide.
2. Their agreement to have their patients participate in our "Patient Care Audit"—an annual national outcomes database completed by patients of participating and non-participating practices to document the improved outcomes associated with this level of patient care.

"Patient Care Excellence" Guidelines Sheet (accompanies disclosure contract)

This sheet outlines a "checklist" of care elements that define "Patient Care Excellence" as it applies to this program. These elements include:

1. **Provider Guarantee:** Patients seen by this practice will receive their care directly by a licensed audiologist, or will have their care supervised and/or overseen by a licensed audiologist.

2. **Assessment:** Patients seen by this practice will receive:

   ■ Auditory Assessment including:
     ■ Comprehensive case history
     ■ Pure-tone, speech, and immittance audiometry
     ■ Measurement of LDL
     ■ Quantification of speech intelligibility in background noise in the unaided condition using a standardized speech-in-noise test.
     ■ Otoscopic inspection and cerumen management
     ■ Determine need for treatment/referral to physician or further testing
     ■ Counsel patient, family, caregivers on the results and recommendations
     ■ Assess candidacy and motivation for amplification
     ■ Determine medical clearance as determined by FDA

   ■ Auditory Needs Assessment
     ■ Identify patient-specific communication needs to determine specific amplification features such as directional mic, noise reduction, DAI, and so forth.
     ■ Complete an objective measurement of the pretreatment hearing handicap. Standardized tests for this purpose include:
       ▪ APHAB
       ▪ COSI
       ▪ HHIE
       ▪ ECHO
       ▪ GHABP
       ▪ International Outcome Inventory-Hearing

   ■ Non-Auditory Needs Assessment
     ■ Determine patient expectations, motivation, assertiveness, manual dexterity, visual acuity, general health, tinnitus condition, occupational demands, presence of support system. Some tools that can be used for this purpose include:
       ▪ COAT
       ▪ Circular Questioning

3. **Hearing Aid Selection:** This practice will select hearing aids/assistive technology based on the results of all three assessment sections above.

4. **Quality Control:** This practice will assess the devices being provided to the patient to insure proper function. Such assessment could include:

    ■ Electroacoustic analysis to ensure instruments meet specifications
    ■ Electroacoustic analysis to insure that the final programmed settings have been documented
    ■ Verification of features functions (electroacoustic or listening) including:
        ▪ Directional mic
        ▪ Noise reduction
        ▪ Feedback management
        ▪ Frequency lowering
        ▪ T-coil
        ▪ FM integration
        ▪ Paired communication
        ▪ Streamer functionality
    ■ Verification of fit, venting, color, and type

5. **Fitting and Verification:** This practice agrees that fitting and verification procedures are viewed as a process that culminates in the optimal fitting. Verification procedures should be based on a validated hearing aid fitting rationale and are expected to yield a comfortable fit of hearing aids including all desired features.

    ■ In the hearing aid fitting process, a signal, preferably speech like, must be presented to the hearing aid microphone as it is worn on the patient's ear with a probe microphone present.
    ■ This result should be compared to a standardized fitting target or goal.
    ■ In the Assistive Technology fiting process, selections must be justified based on need. Assistive technology can be used to address the following if hearing aids alone are judged inadequate based on need:
        ▪ Face-to-face communication

- Broadcast and other electronic media
- Telephone conversation
- Sensitivity to alerting signals and environmental stimuli

6. **Hearing Aid Orientation:** This practice agrees to ensure patients obtained the desired benefits from amplification as easily and efficiently as possible. Hearing aid orientation is complete only when all appropriate information has been provided and the patient/family member/caregiver is competent to handle the instruments or declines further post-fitting care. Orientation should include:

- Care and use instructions
- Insertion and removal practice
- Battery replacement practice
- Telephone use practice
- Wearing schedule with goals and expectations

7. **Counseling and Follow-Up Audiologic Rehabilitation:** This practice agrees to provide patients with a comprehensive understanding of the effects of hearing impairment and to offer strategies to mitigate those effects. Fundamentally, hearing aid fitting is the beginning of the treatment process. A structure that moves the patient to ultimate long-term functionality and acceptance should also be part of overall care. Counseling and rehabilitation strategies should include:

- Anatomy and physiology of the hearing process
- Understanding the audiogram
- Problems associated with speech in noise
- Appropriate/inappropriate communication behaviors
- Communication strategies
- Listening and repair strategies
- Brain exercise strategies
- Ways to control the environment
- Assertive listening training
- Realistic expectations of amplification
- Stress management
- Speechreading skills
- Community resources

8. **Assessing Outcomes:** After long-term treatment goals have been reached, this practice agrees to quantify the impact their treatment strategy has had on overall communication and or quality of life improvement by re-administering handicap surveys and/or speech-in-noise tests utilized in the assessment phase outlined above, and comparing the results of these two sets of tests. Only by measuring the outcomes of treatment can audiologists be assured that interventions make a difference and patients have benefited from their care.

9. **National Outcomes Database:** This practice agrees to enlist their patients to complete a national online survey managed by AuDNet documenting patient perceptions of their care, their outcomes and their satisfaction with treatment. Results of this survey, which is designed to compare patient perceptions of outcomes both for practices participating in this "Patient Care Excellence" program as well as practices that are not, will be shared with AuDNet members and the general public. Below are the questions that will be asked to patients as part of the audit process:

Patient Care Audit Survey

1) When did you purchase your current hearing instrument devices?
2) Had you purchased or worn hearing aids prior to this most current purchase?
3) Was the person who tested your hearing and guided your treatment a licensed audiologist?
4) Prior to recommending treatment, did your audiologist carefully determine your communication needs through questions designed to understand your communication concerns?
5) Did your audiologist assess your hearing using a variety of tests that included your listening to tones and speech?
6) Was your ability to understand speech in the presence of noise tested?
7) Did your audiologist explain your test results and your condition in a satisfactory and understandable way?
8) If present, were others involved in your life included in the discussion of your test results?

9) Did you understand the treatment options that were presented to you so that you felt you were making an informed decision about your treatment?
10) Prior to treatment, did you complete a questionnaire assessing your existing communication abilities?
11) When your hearing instruments were initially fit, did the audiologist measure their performance directly on your ear using a small tube microphone placed in your ear canal?
12) Was the sound you listened to during the above test speech or speech-like?
13) Please rate the instructions you received regarding your use of hearing instruments for each of the following areas:

Patient Care Excellence Discount Program/ Program Participation Agreement

Program Concept: For **AuDNet member audiology practices** who commit to providing all the patient care elements outlined in this agreement, **Unitron Hearing Instruments** will provide an additional 2% discount (on top of the current 30+% discounts currently provided to AuDNet members) on all Unitron products purchased by that AuDNet member practice.

_____(Practice Name)_____ agrees to provide the following patient care elements for its patients:

Check All	Care Element	Description
	Provider Guarantee	This practice agrees that their patients will receive care directly from a licensed audiologist, or will have their care supervised and/or overseen by a licensed audiologist.

Check All	Care Element	Description
	Auditory Assessment	This practice agrees to conduct a complete case history, ear examination, auditory assessment, quantification of hearing difficulty, to refer for medical care when needed, and to explain the results to the patient and significant others present.
	Auditory Needs Assessment	This practice agrees to identify patient-specific communication needs and assess pretreatment communication handicap prior to treatment decision-making.
	Non-Auditory Needs Assessment	This practice agrees to determine patient motivation, dexterity, general health, occupational demands, etc. prior to treatment decision-making.
	Hearing Aid Selection	This practice will select hearing aids/assistive technology based on the results of all three assessment sections above.
	Quality Control	This practice will assess the devices being provided to the patient to ensure proper function.
	Fitting & Verification	This practice agrees to verify hearing aid function on the ear using a probe microphone measurement and comparing that result to a standardized fitting target.
	Hearing Aid Orientation	This practice agrees to ensure patients obtained the desired benefits from amplification as easily and efficiently as possible.
	Counseling & Follow-Up AR	This practice agrees to provide patients with a comprehensive understanding of the effects of hearing impairment and to offer strategies to mitigate those effects.

Check All	Care Element	Description
	Outcome Assessment	This practice agrees to quantify the impact their treatment strategy has had on overall communication and or quality of life improvement by re-administering handicap surveys and/or speech-in-noise tests administered prior to treatment.
	Patient Care Audit	This practice agrees to enlist their patients to complete a national online survey managed by AuDNet documenting patient perceptions of their care, their outcomes and their satisfaction with treatment.

I agree to provide the above patient care elements for the patients treated at this practice.

_____   _____

(Sign) Practice owner or clinic director   Date

_____   _____   _____   _____

City   State   Zip   Phone

AudNet Patient Care Excellence reprinted with permission of AuDNet, Inc.

INDEX